ALEXANDER TECHNIQUE

RICHARD BRENNAN ATI, STAT, is a qualified teacher of the Alexander Technique, as approved by the Society of Teachers of the Alexander Technique. He is a member of Alexander Technique International, a world-wide organisation whose aim is to bring the technique before a greater audience.

Richard Brennan runs a busy Alexander Technique practice in Galway, Ireland, as well as teaching numerous adult education classes and courses throughout the UK and Europe. He also gives talks and lectures at various schools, colleges and universities, for the press and radio, and at health and healing exhibitions. He has been a pioneer in helping to make the technique accessible to many thousands of people. He is currently the Director of the first Alexander Technique Teacher Training College in Ireland.

New Perspectives

THE SERIES

New Perspectives provide attractive and accessible introductions to a comprehensive range of mind, body and spirit topics. Beautifully designed and illustrated, these practical books are written by experts in each subject.

Titles in the series include:

ALEXANDER TECHNIQUE
by Richard Brennan

AROMATHERAPY
by Christine Wildwood

DREAMS
by David Fontana

FENG SHUI
by Man-Ho Kwok with Joanne O'Brien

FLOWER REMEDIES
by Christine Wildwood

HOMEOPATHY
by Peter Adams

MASSAGE
by Stewart Mitchell

MEDITATION
by David Fontana

NLP
by Carol Harris

NUMEROLOGY
by Rodford Barrat

REFLEXOLOGY
by Inge Dougans

TAROT
by A T Mann

New Perspectives

ALEXANDER TECHNIQUE

An Introductory Guide to Natural Poise for Health and Well-Being

RICHARD BRENNAN

ELEMENT

Shaftesbury, Dorset • Boston, Massachusetts
Melbourne, Victoria

© Element Books Limited 1999
Text © Richard Brennan 1991, 1999

First published in 1991 as *Health Essentials:
Alexander Technique* by Element Books Limited

This revised edition first published in Great Britain
in 1999 by Element Books Limited
Shaftesbury, Dorset SP7 8BP

Published in the USA in 1999 by
Element Books, Inc.
160 North Washington Street,
Boston, MA 02114

Published in Australia in 1999 by
Element Books and distributed by
Penguin Australia Limited
487 Maroondah Highway,
Ringwood, Victoria 3134

Designed for Element Books Limited by
Design Revolution, Queens Park Villa,
30 West Drive, Brighton, East Sussex BN2 2GE

ELEMENT BOOKS LIMITED
Editorial Director: Sarah Sutton
Editorial Manager: Jane Pizzey
Commissioning Editor: Grace Cheetham
Production Director: Roger Lane

DESIGN REVOLUTION
Editorial Director: Ian Whitelaw
Art Director: Lindsey Johns
Editor: Kay Macmullan
Designer: Vanessa Good

Printed and bound in Great Britain by
Bemrose Security Printing, Derby

British Library Cataloguing in Publication
data available

Library of Congress Cataloging in Publication
data available

ISBN 1-86204-629-8

CONTENTS

Acknowledgements

I would like to thank the following for their encouragement, inspiration and patience in teaching me the Alexander Technique and in the writing of this book: Cara Brennan, Tim Brennan, Evelyn Burgess, Paul Collins, Margaret Farrar, David Gorman, Trish Hemmingway, Alan Mars, Camilla Mars, Clare Morris, Henry Morris, Jessica Morris, Danny Riley, Refia Sacks, Chris Stevens and many others too numerous to name.

This book is dedicated to all those
who are in pain.

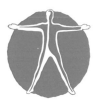

INTRODUCTION

'Know Thyself'
SOCRATES

What do John Cleese, Roald Dahl, Aldous Huxley, Paul Newman, George Bernard Shaw, the Duchess of York and Sting all have in common? 'Not a lot' may be your first thought, and yet they have all spoken of the great benefits that they have received from practising the Alexander Technique.

But why do people of such varied backgrounds and lifestyles all praise the Technique so highly? What benefits have they gained? I shall try to answer these questions at a later stage.

Many people today have heard of the Alexander Technique, and more and more articles in magazines and newspapers discuss it. 'But what is the Alexander Technique exactly?' I hear many people say. There seems to be an air of mystery surrounding it, and this is the very reason why I have written this book.

I hope to present the Technique in such a way that it can be understood by anyone, because I feel that it is everyone's right as a human being to understand themselves more fully. The Alexander Technique has far-reaching consequences in our lives, and not only on a physical level – it can greatly change our mental and emotional outlook on life, too. I suggest that you read through the book and then study each chapter until you feel you have grasped the contents.

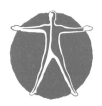

WHAT IS THE ALEXANDER TECHNIQUE?

CHAPTER ONE

Many people believe the Alexander Technique to be a technique of breathing and posture, but this is only a small part of what it really involves. It is, in fact, a method of becoming more aware of ourselves as we go about our everyday activities. As a result we can soon begin to notice, when performing the simplest of tasks, that we may be putting an enormous strain on our bodies without realizing it.

With the help of a teacher the Alexander Technique enables us to let go of many tensions that may have gone unnoticed for months or even years. These tensions are often responsible for aches and pains that accumulate with age. As any doctor will tell you, stress can be the root cause of both physical and mental disease, yet we do little to find out how these tensions first come about.

BAD HABITS

Simply sitting or standing in an unbalanced way will cause certain muscles to be constantly under stress. If these ways of standing and sitting become a habit then, sooner or later, we will have to pay the

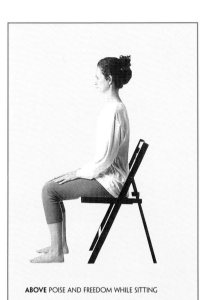

ABOVE POISE AND FREEDOM WHILE SITTING HELPS TO REDUCE MUSCULAR TENSION.

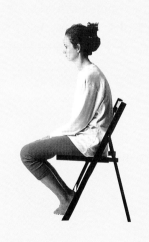

ABOVE HABITUALLY SITTING IN A SLOUCHED POSITION CAN LEAD TO ALL MANNER OF PHYSICAL AND MENTAL DISCOMFORT.

price and sometimes it is a very expensive one indeed.

One of the most common consequences in developed countries is backache, with many millions of sufferers incapacitated every week. Other possible effects of bad posture and mal-coordination are high blood pressure, migraine, asthma, arthritis, depression and insomnia, to name but a few.

TREATMENT

9

Many of our modern methods of dealing with such problems involve the use of powerful drugs to suppress the painful symptoms; these drugs often have unfavourable side effects. We very rarely look for the reason why we have the ailments in the first place. The Alexander Technique can do just this; by putting into practice the principles of the Technique we are able to learn how to move in a balanced and coordinated way so that tensions are not retained in our bodies.

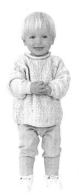

CHILDREN

It is easy to see the natural grace of young children at play; but we slowly start to lose this agility of movement as the pressures of life mould us into our clumsy adult form. By the age of nine or ten the process is often under way, to the extent that I have often treated children as young as ten or eleven for backaches and headaches.

ABOVE CHILDREN MOVE WITH NATURAL GRACE AND POISE, BUT AS THEY GROW OLDER BAD HABITS DEVELOP.

BENEFITS

By moving in a different way we can soon regain ease of movement that had been forgotten; many people report feeling lighter and freer after a course of lessons in the Technique. How we physically feel will directly affect our mental and emotional states, and I often find that people become less irritable and much more at ease with themselves. This can have a rippling effect on those close by, and family and friends alike have remarked on the improved temperament of people who begin to practise the Alexander Technique.

An Alexander Technique lesson consists of two parts:

1 To help the pupil become aware of and let go of excessive muscular tension in the body.

2 To help the pupil find different ways of moving that are easier and more efficient, thus reducing wear and tear on the body.

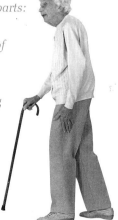

RIGHT THE TECHNIQUE IS FOR PEOPLE OF ANY AGE. THE ELDERLY CAN OFTEN BE HELPED TO OVERCOME PROBLEMS WITH ARTHRITIS.

10

YOUR FIRST ALEXANDER TECHNIQUE LESSON

At first you may be asked to lie face up on a table; there will be no need to remove your clothes apart from your shoes. The teacher may then ask you neither to resist nor help while he gently moves your head and limbs. It never hurts, as is sometimes the case in other therapies, since the movements are often very slow and gentle. When the teacher finds some resistance due to muscular tension, he or she will then ask you to release the tension in the affected muscles; he or she may suggest ways to help you to do this. At the end of a half-hour session, the difference in how you feel may well be quite dramatic. You may feel much lighter, as gravity will be working on you in a very different way. Sometimes, even long-standing aches and pains have been known to disappear completely, much to the pupil's amazement.

The teacher will often then take you through a series of movements in order to find out when you are tensing your muscles unnecessarily. You will explore new, more naturally coordinated, ways of moving. This will produce a greater sense of well-being and you may well have more energy left to do the things you want to, instead of collapsing in front of the television. Have you ever wondered where children get all their energy from? It is often that their actions are much more efficient than ours and therefore they still have lots of energy left when we feel exhausted.

LEFT YOUR FIRST LESSON WITH AN ALEXANDER TECHNIQUE TEACHER WILL INVOLVE THE GENTLE MOVEMENT OF YOUR HEAD AND LIMBS.

11

The Alexander Technique is referred to as a re-education rather than a therapy, because the practitioner is teaching you how to help yourself. If any ailment or illness is cured in the process then it will be you that is curing yourself.

Although the effects of the Technique can be far reaching it is, at the same time, simple and easily understood. The important qualities to have are patience and a willingness to learn about oneself. In some cases people find it hard at first to grasp some of the basic principles because they are looking for something more complicated.

MUSIC AND SPORT

If you play a musical instrument or are involved in a sport of any kind then the Technique will be especially helpful as it will increase your ability to perform for longer without the usual tensions. Many of the major music and drama colleges have resident Alexander teachers because they have found that many students are forced to give up their careers due to chronic tensions that arise from the way they hold their bodies while performing. Not only have a great many students reported feeling much better, but they also say it has improved their performances. In the case of professional sportsmen and women in every field, the Alexander Technique has also proved all important when trying to break world records.

LEFT AS WELL AS BEING GOOD FOR YOUR BODY AND MIND, THE ALEXANDER TECHNIQUE CAN ALSO IMPROVE MUSICAL PERFORMANCE.

HOW IS THE
ALEXANDER TECHNIQUE DIFFERENT?

The Alexander Technique is often grouped with various forms of complementary medicines, but it stands in its own right, being quite unique. This is because it gives each and every one of us the responsibility for our own well-being. We are encouraged to think for ourselves, so it is a useful tool for awareness and self-development.

When we begin to apply the principles of the Alexander Technique in our lives, we see that we are not learning anything new; rather, we are unlearning. Alexander was often quoted as saying:

'If you stop doing the wrong things the right thing will happen automatically.'

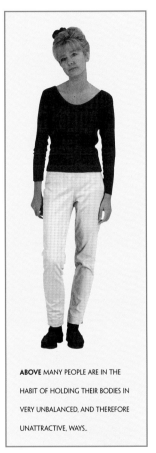

ABOVE MANY PEOPLE ARE IN THE HABIT OF HOLDING THEIR BODIES IN VERY UNBALANCED, AND THEREFORE UNATTRACTIVE, WAYS..

13

It really does not matter what age you are (I have taught people ranging in age from 5 to 84), you can still regain much of the poise and grace that you once had in childhood. If you do not believe me, just go and have a lesson and see for yourself.

It is astonishing how many of us grossly interfere with the way that our bodies work. Just look around the next time you are waiting in a queue at the supermarket or the bank, and you are bound to see people who have hunched shoulders or arched backs. Many of them will not even be standing up straight; they will be standing on one leg or leaning backwards at quite an angle.

They will, of course, be totally unaware that they are distorting their bodies, and that these distortions will become more acute with age. This is because over the years we develop many habits that feel 'comfortable' even though they may be putting a strain on our bodies.

We rarely give much thought to ourselves apart from how we look. We may spend many hours and hundreds of pounds improving our appearance and striving to look younger. Yet, what is more attractive and youthful than someone who moves with grace and poise?

So, as you can see, there are many benefits in applying the Technique in your life. You may just wish to use it as a prevention against future ill-health – you do not need to have anything wrong with you in order to benefit from Alexander lessons. It is widely agreed that prevention is better than cure, but how many people really take steps in order to ensure good health in later life?

14

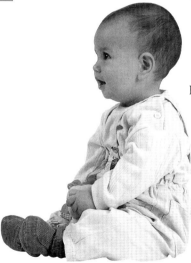

I am naturally biased, being a teacher of the Alexander Technique, but I cannot help thinking that if some of the basic principles were taught in our schools then perhaps millions of people would not suffer so greatly later on in life.

Being aware of one's body is nothing new. People involved with the martial arts have realized the importance for many thousands of years. They too understand that the mind can have a marked effect upon how one moves.

ABOVE THE ALEXANDER TECHNIQUE HELPS US TO RELEARN THE
NATURAL POISE THAT WE WERE ALL BLESSED WITH AT BIRTH.

A THERAPY OR AN EDUCATION?

Many people think that the Alexander Technique is another therapy similar to homeopathy, osteopathy and acupuncture. It is very different, however, because it centres around the pupil consciously letting go of his or her own tension. The effects of Alexander's work may be, and very often are, therapeutic, but it is much more a process by which pupils learn how they can help themselves. The pupil takes an active part in the process and the teacher cannot do anything without his or her willingness.

Once we can find the reason for our aches or pains then it often does not take long to put things right. Alexander once said,

'You can change the habit of a lifetime in a few moments,
if you just use your brains.'

I personally have been a witness to this time and time again, and have been very surprised at how quickly many people have changed once they have realized the reason for their problem.

Many of our common actions, like sitting, standing or walking, have to be learned all over again and these new movements may, at first, feel very strange. The way in which we are used to moving may be the very cause of many tensions within our body. These tensions often lead to sickness or pain, but the movements that cause them may feel completely normal.

As these tensions in our bodies cause us pain we then become even more tense, and so a vicious cycle is set up. If we can start to learn how to use our bodies in a different way then the muscular tension often slowly disappears.

These different ways of moving are not new to us, they are the ways we moved as children – but we have forgotten them. I therefore call the Alexander Technique a method of re-education, a way of re-discovering the natural grace of movement that we were all born with.

If you do decide to have a course of lessons then it is important to realize that this re-education does take time and it is sometimes hard to understand what is happening for the first six or seven lessons. Eventually, however, you will have learned a technique that you can use to help yourself for the rest of your life.

There is nothing like pain to motivate people into looking at themselves, but if people do come for lessons before the tensions or pain are too bad, then often they may not need so many lessons. The main qualities to have in this process of change are an open mind and a willingness to look at oneself.

MIND, BODY AND SPIRIT UNITY

F. M. Alexander (1869–1955), the founder of the Technique was convinced that the mind, body and spirit were inseparable. In other words, the way we think will directly affect the way we feel and can often be at the bottom of many tensions or diseases. Similarly, the way in which we sit or stand will alter the way in which we feel or think.

This can easily be seen in a person suffering from depression – they will often sit in a slumped manner with rounded shoulders and a collapsed chest. This posture will interfere with their breathing and, ultimately, with the body's life energy. Whenever this person needs to move there has to be an enormous amount of effort to bring them out of their slumped posture, so

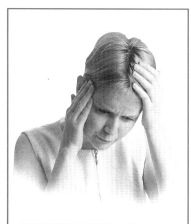

ABOVE MANY OF OUR PROBLEMS, BOTH PHYSICAL AND MENTAL, CAN STEM FROM THE WAY IN WHICH WE MOVE OR HOLD OUR BODIES.

most of the time they cannot be bothered to perform even simple tasks. This will only add to their reasons for being depressed, and so they enter a vicious cycle.

Changing the way in which we think is as much a part of the Alexander Technique as changing the way in which we move. The Technique is a way of using our minds to direct our bodies in order to keep them as stress-free as possible. This, in turn, will allow the natural healing processes to function as effectively as possible.

Muscle tension that has been allowed to build up unnoticed over many years will interfere with the circulatory, respiratory and nervous systems. This can eventually lead to many of the illnesses that we see today, most of which could have been avoided altogether. These tensions are merely a reflection of the stressed condition of our minds.

CHOICE

We are trained from an early age to be goal-orientated or, as Alexander described it, 'end gain'. Maybe we should ask ourselves if we are human *beings* or human *doers*? Due to our modern civilization I fear that many of us are becoming the latter. How many of us stop just for a moment and ask ourselves,

'Am I doing what I really want to do with my life or am I finding that I have little or no choice in the matter?'

The Alexander Technique is about having free choice on every level, about living, and not just surviving. We seem to be living in a rat-race, yet it is important to remember that it does not matter who wins, that person is still a rat. Alexander believed that man had a right to knowledge and awareness, and that his Technique could be the next stage in our evolutionary development. He also recognized that most of the time we are held back by time and fear. We spend most of our time performing actions for others, rather than doing what we really want to do. He once said,

Everyone wants to change and yet remain the same.

So we also have to be prepared to change our way of thinking if we are ever to free our bodies from stresses and strains. The benefits are enormous. We have so much to gain and so little to lose; a willingness to learn about ourselves is the only essential requirement. Once we are able to let go of the tensions that are holding back both mind and body, then we will begin to experience the joy of life that we once had as children.

18

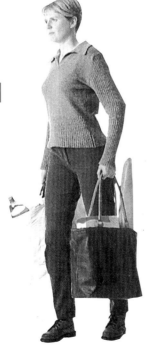

ABOVE IN ORDER TO CHANGE THE WAY THAT WE MOVE, WE MUST FIRST BECOME AWARE OF THE WAY THAT WE REACT IN EVERYDAY SITUATIONS.

AWARENESS

The first step to take when learning the Alexander Technique is to try to become more aware of yourself, how you go about your activities as well as what you are thinking as you do them. This is quite hard at first, but gets easier with practice. Later on in this book you will find exercises that will help you to increase your awareness while performing common everyday actions.

You may discover that a 'comfortable' habit of standing or sitting is very stressful. Have you ever caught sight of yourself in a shop window or on a video, and got a shock because you did not know that you moved like that? It is often such an experience that motivates the starting of Alexander lessons because a person sees that if he or she continues in the same way there could be serious problems later on in life.

Pain is the other main reason why many people are forced to look at themselves, yet the signs of tension may well have been present for many years. Most of us are too busy with our lives to even notice tension and we are often taken by surprise when our body starts to let us down. If we learn to become more aware of ourselves then we may well be able to avoid many ailments later on in life.

Most of the time many of us are thinking about anything but the task at hand. The Alexander Technique is a very practical method that enables us to be conscious of each moment; this enhances the quality of our life and enables us to live life to the full.

TIME AS A CAUSE OF TENSION

If there is one factor more responsible for tension than any other, it is probably time. Our civilization is ruled by it.

From the age of five when we first start school, we are under a pressure to be at certain places at certain times. It is obvious, standing outside the school gates at nine o'clock every day, that parents are already feeling stress and anxiety as a result of getting their children ready on time.

As children, we live in another world, a world ruled by the five senses. A child will naturally be drawn to attractive things that he sees or hears. But as adults we usually have a plan of what our day is going to be like and, if we get behind in our schedule, then we tend to become tense.

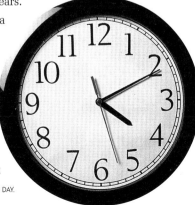

RIGHT OUR LIVES ARE DOMINATED BY TIME – THINK HOW MANY TIMES YOU LOOK AT A CLOCK OR WATCH DURING THE DAY.

SIMPLE TIPS FOR REDUCING STRESS

Many people will argue that we have to live within these time structures unless we drop out of society; this may be true but there is much we can do to alleviate stress:

1. Leave plenty of time to get where you are going. This is especially important when hold-ups are possible, such as in heavy traffic or at road-works.

2. Try not to take on too much. Most of us find it hard to say no to friends or colleagues and we then take on more than we can manage; this causes an incredible amount of tension as we rush around trying to get all our jobs finished before the deadlines that we have set for ourselves. It is a good idea to say, 'Yes – if I have the time', rather than commit to something that may not be possible.

3. If you are unavoidably delayed try to phone and let people know what has happened. This is obvious advice but it is often the obvious that we forget.

4. If you are behind schedule and there is nothing you can do about it – RELAX. This is easier said than done, but it is very important. Tense and irritated drivers who are late for work often cause accidents. It is always when we are rushing that we knock the milk over or forget to turn off the iron, which causes us to be later still.

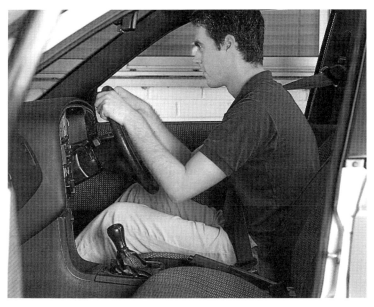

ABOVE MANY CAR ACCIDENTS COULD BE PREVENTED IF DRIVERS WERE MORE AWARE.

When I started having Alexander lessons I noticed that when I was late for an appointment, which was quite often, I started to tense my neck muscles and poke my head forward as though this would get me there sooner. These circumstances had always brought on neck tension, but I had not noticed it before. This tension remained in my body even after I had reached my destination, and it eventually caused headaches, neck problems and a general lack of coordination.

Tensions stay in our body without us even realizing, and we only become aware of them years later when they show themselves in the form of arthritis or backpain.

In order to practise the Alexander Technique you will need to give yourself time to observe how you use your body, but this does not mean you have to do things slowly. Just give yourself a moment or two before acting to find the easiest and most efficient way of going about it. In the end you will save yourself time.

Alexander called this process of stopping and thinking about actions before carrying them out INHIBITION. This should not be confused with the term used by Freud to mean suppressing or holding back feelings. In chapter 4 we will look at inhibition in detail.

FEAR AS A CAUSE OF TENSION

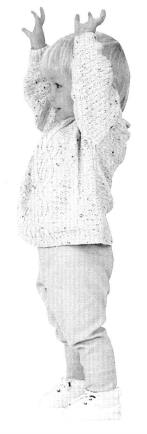

Fear is the other main factor that can cause tension within our bodies.

FEAR OF FALLING

Children are always falling over and they rarely seem to hurt themselves yet, as we get older, one fall can put us out of action for months. Why is this?

As we get older our muscles grow more and more tense; when we fall, the fear makes us tense our muscles until we are rigid, this then makes us more vulnerable to breaking bones.

An interesting fact is that many hip operations, as a result of falling, are caused by muscle tension breaking the hip before the person has even reached the ground. The reason why people who faint or who fall over when drunk do not hurt themselves is because their muscles are relaxed.

ABOVE BECAUSE THEIR MUSCLES ARE MORE RELAXED THAN ADULTS', CHILDREN RARELY SERIOUSLY INJURE THEMSELVES WHEN THEY FALL.

FEAR OF CRITICISM

One can easily see the muscle tension that is present when children are being told off, and their whole posture changes as a result; if this happens often enough at school or at home then these tensions can easily become fixed in their bodies.

The list of fears is a long one, from the fear of losing one's job to the fear of death, and each one will cause stress within our bodies without us even realizing it. We are often completely unaware of many of the fears that we are suffering from.

The Alexander Technique can help to release much of this muscular tension before it is able to do real, or even irreversible, damage. We only have this one body, so the way in which we use it is of the utmost importance. It is often the case that we look after our house and our car better than we look after ourselves, but both our house and our car can be replaced – our bodies cannot.

'The true miracle is not to fly in the air,
or to walk on water,
but to walk on this earth.'

CHINESE PROVERB

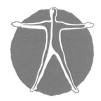

THE HISTORY OF THE ALEXANDER TECHNIQUE

CHAPTER TWO

Frederick Matthias Alexander, the founder of the Alexander Technique, was born in Australia on 20 January 1869. Alexander (or FM as his friends used to call him) was born prematurely and was not expected to live more than a few weeks. He only survived due to his mother's love and care.

Alexander was plagued with one illness after another throughout his childhood, mainly suffering from asthma and other breathing problems. As a result, he had to be taken away from school and was given private tuition in the evenings from the local school teacher.

This left plenty of free time during the day, which he spent with his father's horses; he gradually became an expert at training and managing them. At this time he acquired his sensitivity of touch, which proved to be invaluable later in his career.

At the age of eleven his health slowly began to improve; by the time he was seventeen financial hardship within the family forced Alexander to leave the outdoor life that he had grown to love so much. He began work in the office of a tin-mining company at the nearby town of Mount Bischoff. In his spare time he became more and more interested in amateur dramatics, as well as teaching himself to play the violin. After three years he had saved up enough money to travel to Melbourne where he stayed with his uncle. During the next three months Alexander spent all his hard-earned money visiting the theatre, art galleries or going to concerts. He had decided to train to be a reciter.

He then took various jobs including that of a clerk to an estate agent, a shop assistant in a department store and even as a tea taster for a firm of tea merchants. This paid for his training, which he did in the evenings and at weekends. Alexander very quickly established an excellent reputation as an actor and reciter and soon formed his own theatre company, which specialized in one-man Shakespearean recitals.

VOICE PROBLEMS

All went well for a short while, but then his childhood respiratory problems returned. His voice became hoarse and the audience began to notice that he was sucking in air loudly between sentences.

On one occasion Alexander completely lost his voice during one of his performances. This was a great blow to his confidence and he began to turn down work for fear of losing his voice in front of an audience.

He became desperate and was willing to try anything in order to solve his problem. Alexander sought the advice of numerous doctors and voice trainers who gave him different medicines or voice exercises, but this only brought him temporary relief.

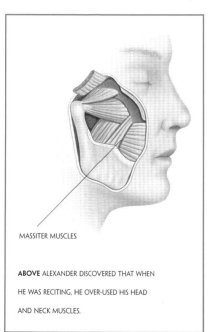

MASSITER MUSCLES

ABOVE ALEXANDER DISCOVERED THAT WHEN HE WAS RECITING, HE OVER-USED HIS HEAD AND NECK MUSCLES.

Finally, one of the doctors who had been advising him prescribed complete rest of the voice for a full two weeks before his next recital. Alexander, being a very determined man, hardly uttered a word for the next two weeks.

At the beginning of his next performance his voice was crystal clear, but half an hour later the hoarseness reappeared. By the end of the evening the problem had returned and he was hardly able to speak.

Alexander was bitterly disappointed. He thought his voice would never be permanently healed. He believed that he would have to give up a career to which he was deeply committed and which had promised to be highly successful.

The very next day he went back to the doctor to tell him what had happened. The doctor then told Alexander that he must go on with the treatment. Alexander could see no point at all in doing this and flatly refused. He believed that if his voice had been alright at the beginning of his performance, and yet he could hardly speak by the end, then it must be a result of something that he was doing while reciting that was causing the problem.

Alexander left the surgery determined that he would find out the solution to his curious problem. He did exactly that, little knowing that he was about to stumble upon one of the greatest discoveries of this century.

SEARCHING FOR A CAUSE

It is important to remember that it was Alexander's all-consuming passion for the theatre that gave him the determination to find out the

FIRST DISCOVERIES

After Alexander's conversation with his doctor he was left with only two leads:

1. When he rested his voice, or only spoke normally, then the hoarseness disappeared.
2. When he began to project his voice during recitals then the hoarseness always returned.

He began to experiment on himself. He started to speak and then to recite in front of a mirror. After a short while Alexander noticed that he was doing three things while reciting that did not seem to do when he was using his normal speaking voice:

1. He tended to pull his head back and down onto his spine.
2. He pressed down his larynx (or windpipe), the site of the vocal cords.
3. He began to suck in air through his mouth, producing a gasping sound.

27

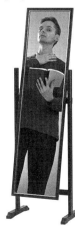

LEFT ONLY BY CAREFULLY MONITORING HIS MOVEMENTS IN A MIRROR, COULD ALEXANDER SEE HOW HE LOST HIS VOICE DURING HIS RECITALS.

cause of his hoarseness. He was faced with one setback after another, as we shall see, and most people would have given up along the way. It took him seven long and difficult years to find out where he was going wrong.

After many months of careful observation he realized that he was in fact doing exactly the same thing while talking. His actions were not so obvious when talking, however, so he had never noticed this habit. He had been using a great deal of unnecessary tension when reciting. This tension was the root cause of his problem.

When Alexander came to correct his problem, however, he began to experience great difficulties. While still using the mirror he tried not to tense his neck muscles, nor to press down his larynx, nor to make the gasping sounds. He found that he was unable to do anything to improve the condition of his larynx or his breathing, but he was able to stop pulling his head back. This suggested to him that the tension in his neck was causing the other two problems.

28

THE PRIMARY CONTROL

Alexander's discovery of the Primary Control was the first important stage in his investigation. The Primary Control acts as the main organizer in the body. It is situated in the area of the neck and governs all our movements, both voluntary and involuntary. The Primary Control is often referred to as 'the head, neck, back relationship'.

It is essential to point out that this relationship is not one of position, but one of freedom. When muscle tension interferes with this relationship, the rest of the body is affected. The body begins to lose coordination and balance, and starts to move less efficiently. A good example of this can be seen in riding. When a rider wishes to stop a horse in an emergency, he, or she, pulls the horse's head back by use of the reins. The animal immediately loses its coordination and soon comes to a stop.

It is also worth noting that it is very difficult to tell when we are tensing our neck muscles and when we are not, and this is perhaps why Alexander had been unaware of the tension in this neck before.

TENSION LEADS TO MORE TENSION

Having discovered the Primary Control, Alexander then noticed that when he released the tension in his neck muscles, the hoarseness in his voice started to disappear. Doctors who examined him, told him that his throat and vocal cords had started to improve. This showed that the way he used his muscles when reciting had a marked effect on his voice and breathing.

Alexander went on to notice that, when he pulled his head back, he also tended to lift his chest and make his whole body shorter. He also found that he was arching and narrowing his back.

He therefore realized that the tension in his neck was causing tensions throughout his whole body.

FAULTY SENSORY PERCEPTION

Alexander started to examine the effects that shortening and lengthening of his body had on his voice. He discovered that the hoarseness came back only when he pulled his head back and down onto his spine and so shortened his stature. All he had to do was to put his head forward and up, instead of pulling it back and down, and his problem would be solved.

When he looked in the mirror, however, he saw that when he put his head forward, he was still lifting his chest and arching his back. He could hardly believe his eyes.

Alexander then placed two extra mirrors either side of the original mirror that he had been using. He quickly noticed that, although he had been convinced that he was putting his head forward, he was in fact pulling his head back with even more tension than before. When he felt that he was doing one thing, in fact, he was really doing the opposite. Alexander called this faulty sensory perception. Originally he thought this was a problem that he alone suffered from, but he later discovered that nearly everyone suffers in the same way.

As he continued to experiment, he began to notice more tensions in his legs, feet and even his toes. His toes were pulled in and bent downward so that his feet were very arched. This threw his weight onto the outside of the feet, affecting his whole balance and causing stress throughout his whole body.

Slowly Alexander realized that the tension that he had first noticed was not of particular parts of his body, but of his whole being. He was still convinced that if he could somehow get rid of the tension in the neck then the other problems would automatically be solved. He stopped all his experimentation and considered what he had learnt so far:

FURTHER DISCOVERIES

1. The fact that he was pulling his head back and down, when he thought he was putting it forward and up, proved that he could no longer trust the messages that his body was sending to his brain.

2. He had no control over the messages that his body was giving him.

3. This faulty sensory perception, as he called it, was a habit.

4. This habit was accentuated by reciting.

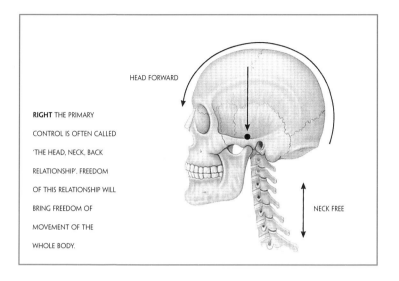

HEAD FORWARD

RIGHT THE PRIMARY
CONTROL IS OFTEN CALLED
'THE HEAD, NECK, BACK
RELATIONSHIP'. FREEDOM
OF THIS RELATIONSHIP WILL
BRING FREEDOM OF
MOVEMENT OF THE
WHOLE BODY.

NECK FREE

DIRECTIONS

31

Alexander started to direct his own actions by inventing orders that he gave to himself when standing, sitting and reciting. He called these orders 'directions'. The main three were:

1. **Allow the neck to be free.**

2. **Allow the head to go forward and upward.**

3. **Allow the back to lengthen and widen.**

These directions were opposite to his old habits and successfully brought about the change that he had been seeking.

He did have one last setback, however; as long as he was not reciting he was free from tension in the neck but, as soon as he began to use his voice, all his old habits returned. It seemed to him that he had come so far in discovering so much about his problem but was unable to bring about any real change.

INHIBITION

Alexander was thoroughly fed up and gave up trying to 'do' anything to reach his goal. To his amazement, the very results that he had been after for several years were achieved. At last he saw that, if he was ever to get rid of his old habits, then he must refuse to do anything at all until he had given himself the directions. Alexander called this 'inhibition'.

As previously mentioned, this is not the type of inhibition talked of in Freudian books, which means to hold back feelings. Inhibition, as recommended by Alexander, is the ability to pause for a moment until we are ready to carry out an action properly. A good example of this is a cat. A cat inhibits its desire to chase a bird until it is ready so that it has the highest chance of success.

So Alexander worked out a technique that not only freed him from the tendency which was at the bottom of his vocal troubles, but also cured his asthma from which he had suffered from birth.

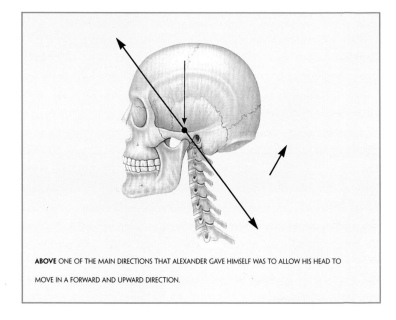

ABOVE ONE OF THE MAIN DIRECTIONS THAT ALEXANDER GAVE HIMSELF WAS TO ALLOW HIS HEAD TO MOVE IN A FORWARD AND UPWARD DIRECTION.

TEACHING OTHERS

Alexander then returned to his much loved reciting career. By this time there was a great interest in how he had overcome his voice problem when so many other treatments had failed. He soon found himself teaching what he had learned to fellow actors who had similar problems.

Before long many people from all over the world had heard about Alexander's successes, and doctors and specialists began to send him some of their patients. Within a few months he was teaching full-time.

ALBERT REDDEN ALEXANDER

As he became more busy, he asked his brother, Albert Redden Alexander (nicknamed AR for short) to join him. Frederick quickly taught his brother the Technique and they worked side by side, often having long discussions about their work and making changes to the Technique as they went along.

MOVE TO LONDON

In 1903 J. W. Stewart McKay, a prominent surgeon in Sydney, persuaded Alexander to go to London so that he could bring his valuable Technique before the world. So in the spring of 1904 he left Australia, never to return.

He arrived in London some months later with letters of introduction to both actors and physicians. He was soon joined by his brother and the two of them set up a practice in the Army and Navy Mansions on Victoria Street. As in Australia, they were soon working flat out with people coming to them from all walks of life. Many of the leading actors of that day came to him and some of them, such as Sir Henry Irving, used to have his professional help between acts of their plays. Apart from several trips to teach in the USA during the war years, Alexander spent the rest of his life teaching his Technique in London.

PUBLICATIONS

Between 1906 and 1908 Alexander published pamphlets and articles, both privately and in the press, and in 1910 his first book, entitled *Man's Supreme Inheritance*, was published. At the beginning of the First World War he sailed for the United States of America and spent the next ten years dividing his teaching between there and England. He continued to write, publishing a further two books entitled *Conscious Control* and *Constructive Conscious Control*.

FAMILY LIFE

In 1920 Alexander married the actress Edith Page, a fellow Australian, but his marriage was not particularly happy and for most of the time they lived apart. She did not believe in his work, yet it is reported that he always treated her with affection. After a couple of years they adopted a child, whom they named Peggy, of whom he was very fond.

ALEXANDER TECHNIQUE SCHOOL

In the mid 1920s a class was set up in London; in 1934 this became a school at Penhill in Kent. His Technique was practised throughout the school. Alexander saw that since most problems start in early life it should be possible to avoid these with the right teaching. By learning his Technique children became more upright and were eager to learn. He was well pleased with the success of the school and was convinced that these children were most successful in learning other subjects as a result of his Technique.

When Alexander reached the age of sixty he was persuaded by many friends, afraid that his most valuable secrets would die with him, to set up a training school to teach others to be teachers of his Technique. So, in 1931, he began to train teachers to carry on his work; this school was set up in his home at 16 Ashley Place in London SW1 and it continued up to his death in October 1955.

RECOGNITION

Throughout his life Alexander tried to get his work recognized by the medical profession, but with little success, even though the *British Medical Journal* wrote of his Technique in 1930:

> '*Mr. Alexander's work is of first class importance and investigation by the medical profession is imperative.*'

Again, in 1937, nineteen doctors published a letter in the *BMJ* stating that they believed, through personal experience, that Alexander's teaching was very beneficial in the cure and prevention of many diseases. They called upon the medical profession to investigate his claims and to include the Alexander Technique in the training of doctors. Unfortunately for many millions of people, nothing was ever done about either of these suggestions.

The Nobel prize winners Nikolaas Tinbergen and Sir Charles Sherrington praised Alexander's work; Nikolaas Tinbergen even dedicated his prize-winning speech to Alexander, but even to this day Alexander has not really received the recognition he so richly deserves. Among his many pupils were the authors George Bernard Shaw and Aldous Huxley, the scientists Professor Raymond Dart, Professor George E. Coghill and Professor Frank Pierce Jones, as well as many well-known actors – too numerous to list in full.

Today there are thousands of trained teachers throughout the world carrying on his work over forty years after his death. The numbers are growing as the demand ever increases.

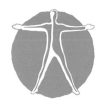

WHAT CAN THE TECHNIQUE DO FOR YOU?

CHAPTER THREE

You may be one of those millions of people suffering from backache, stiff neck, headaches, arthritis or other symptoms for which there seems to be no cure. Although the Alexander Technique does not set out to cure specific problems, it does help to uncover and change those harmful habits that, although we may be unaware of them, are often the underlying cause of a problem.

You may be suffering from stress as a result of work or other circumstances. The Technique will help you to look more closely at your reactions in everyday situations and will enable you to see clearly for yourself how, without realizing it, you add to the build-up of tension in your life. When you are made aware of this you can make the choice not to react in a stressed way and you will therefore be able to remain calm even when your life becomes hectic.

If you are a musician, an actor, a dancer, a singer or a sports person you rely on your body being in the very best shape in order to

ABOVE CHANGING THE WAY WE USE OUR BODIES CAN BRING A REDUCTION IN TENSION AND IN STRESS-RELATED PROBLEMS.

obtain the best results. The Alexander Technique, by helping you to release the build-up of tension, helps you to perform to your maximum ability with the minimum amount of effort.

Lastly, you may be perfectly healthy but are one of the increasing number of people who want to take responsibility for their own well-being and wish to discover more about themselves. You can use the Alexander Technique to prevent future problems: after all, prevention is better than cure.

These are only a few of the ways that the Technique can help people. It can be used by anyone to improve whatever it is that is important to him or her. The only requirements are patience, a willingness to learn and a readiness to let go of the habits of a lifetime.

HABITS

We all have habits that we are aware of, but the habits that Alexander referred to are below our level of consciousness. In other words, we are completely unaware of them, usually because our mind is somewhere else.

At any given moment our mind may wander into the future or into the past; in fact many of us are very rarely present in the here and now. Alexander often referred to this condition as the 'mind-wandering habit', which will often lead us to use our bodies in a very uncoordinated way, without even realizing it.

ABOVE DETRIMENTAL HABITS, SUCH AS SITTING WITH THE LEGS CROSSED, ARE VERY COMMON.

Have you ever been walking or driving somewhere and completely missed your turning because your mind was somewhere else? I am sure the answer is yes; we all do it from time to time. Every day, we are preoccupied with thoughts without even noticing it. While this is happening we may unconsciously be standing, walking or sitting in ways that are a strain on the body.

If we do this often enough, and many of us do, we get into the habit of behaving in a particular way and eventually the muscle tension that is required for these unnatural positions becomes fixed into our body. Very soon these fixed positions start to restrict our movement and by the time we reach old age many of us struggle to get around.

Much of this stiffness is avoidable if we act early enough and, through having Alexander lessons, we can learn to move in different ways.

RELEASING TENSION

First we should understand that the tightness in one set of muscles will affect the balance of our whole body. After releasing this tension, we will find that movements become easier and we experience a sense of lightness that perhaps we may not have felt since childhood. We begin to perform activities with greater efficiency and therefore have much more energy at the end of the day.

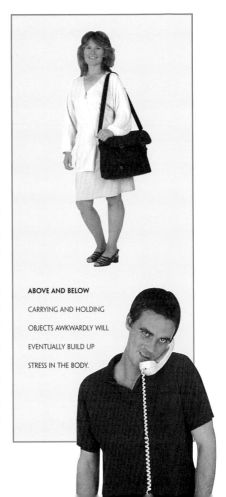

ABOVE AND BELOW

CARRYING AND HOLDING OBJECTS AWKWARDLY WILL EVENTUALLY BUILD UP STRESS IN THE BODY.

38

The same effects may be achieved by having a massage but, unlike a massage, the feeling of lightness may last for days and we can eventually learn how to release tension for ourselves.

FEELINGS

An important part of Alexander's discovery was that our physical, emotional and mental states are all related, so it follows that the way in which we use our bodies will, in turn, alter the way in which we think and how we feel. Unhappiness and feelings of unfulfillment, therefore, must stem from the way in which we move in this world. By practising the Alexander Technique feelings and thoughts can begin to change. Alexander wrote on the subject of unhappiness:

'I shall now endeavour to show that the lack of real happiness manifested by the majority of adults today is due to the fact that they are experiencing, not an improving, but a continually deteriorating use of their psycho-physical selves. This is associated with those defects, imperfections, undesirable traits of character, disposition, temperament, etc., characteristic of imperfectly coordinated people struggling through life beset with certain maladjustments of the psycho-physical organism, which are actually setting up conditions of irritation and pressure during both sleeping and waking hours. Whilst the maladjustments remain present, these malconditions increase day by day and week by week, and foster that unsatisfactory state which we call "Unhappiness".'

39

RIGHT FREEDOM OF THE BODY IS REFLECTED BY THE HAPPINESS AND ALERTNESS THAT YOUNG CHILDREN POSSESS.

In short, the habitual way of being that so may of us are encouraged to fall into from a very early age is bound to affect our physical, mental and even our spiritual well-being. This will encourage undesirable qualitites such as frustration, anger, lack of confidence and a general feeling of dissatisfaction with life in general. These states will, in turn, begin to become habitual.

Nobody begins life feeling angry or frustrated, no one as an infant is dissatisfied or lacks self-esteem. These are things that we begin to feel as life's pressures take their toll on us.

Every experience that we have creates muscular tension in our body. The trouble is that we forget to let go of the tension. Animals also feel these tensions, but they instinctively know how to relax after they have completed an action.

So the Alexander Technique not only helps to improve posture and coordination, it also balances emotions and helps to bring us peace of mind.

Later on in this chapter you will see how it has helped specific people in their lives, but first I would like to show how the Technique can help some of the more common ailments that many people suffer today.

BACKACHE

An estimated one million people are off work with back pain each week in the UK alone. This figure does not include school children, students, housewives, mothers with small children, senior citizens, or people who are unemployed; nor does it include those many people who struggle into work with an aching back. The cost to industry of this absence from work is estimated to be over £250,000,000 each year, to say nothing of the individual's suffering or loss of income. Much of this is completely avoidable. By having Alexander lessons, many people would be able to learn how to sit, stand or move so that they do not put so much strain on the back muscles, often bringing instant relief to their back (see chapter 6).

STIFF NECK OR FROZEN SHOULDERS

This again can be entirely due to excess muscle tension and, with the help of a teacher, the pupil can learn to relax the muscles that are causing the problem.

HYPERTENSION

High blood pressure, or hypertension, is a very common problem. Many of the arteries and veins of the circulation system run through the muscles of the body. If these muscles are always tensed, then they become hardened; this may restrict the flow of blood to and from the heart. The heart has then got to work harder and harder to keep the flow of blood going, thus causing high blood pressure.

Chris Stevens, a physicist and Alexander teacher, has performed experiments on people suffering from hypertension and has shown that Alexander lessons can lower blood pressure significantly.

41

HEADACHES AND MIGRAINE

While working on people who suffer from these conditions I have always found that the neck muscles are extremely tight. With headaches the pain will almost always disappear (while I am working on them) as soon as they release the tension that has caused the pain. With migraines, I often find that results take longer, but the attacks often become less frequent and their intensity decreases after a course of lessons.

ASTHMA

Alexander himself suffered from asthma very badly as a child, but after developing his Technique he freed himself from respiratory problems for the rest of his life. Many pupils who have come to me have been dramatically helped by learning the Technique.

ARTHRITIS

Arthritis is yet another very common illness in today's society. It is most common in older people and it is often believed that there is no cure because it is a sign that the body is wearing out. Most people are just given pain-killers to cope with the condition. What is often happening is that two bones in the body are being pulled together by muscle tension, which can cause wear and tear. Once the pressure is reduced then the bones can heal themselves because bone is, like everything in the body, a living tissue.

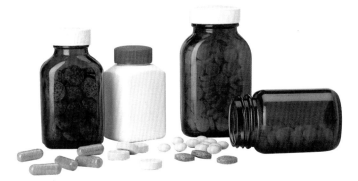

ABOVE DRUGS CANNOT DEAL WITH UNDERLYING CAUSES OF DEPRESSION.

DEPRESSION

Depression is often treated with powerful drugs that have many side effects. Although these drugs do have their place and many people gain relief from them, they do not usually solve the problem. When someone is depressed, it is often obvious from their body shape. If you can alter the shape by relaxing the muscles, then the mental and emotional condition of the person will also change.

BREATHING AND VOICE

In order to treat breathing difficulties certain muscles need to be relaxed in order to free the rib-cage; the breathing will then automatically start to work naturally. As Alexander was often heard to say – if you stop doing the wrong thing, then the right thing will emerge naturally.

There are so many illnesses that can be helped by the Alexander Technique because, whatever problem we may have, the remedy is always the same: find out what it is that is causing the problem, stop doing whatever it is and then you will soon start to feel better. This may seem very simple but, in my experience, I have seen it work time and time again. I myself have often been surprised at how quickly so many people feel the benefit of the Alexander Technique

Learning about our bodies and how they work is obviously a good thing. It is important to remember, however, that the Alexander Technique is not a treatment or a cure – you have to take an active part in the process. You will be curing yourself.

43

CASE HISTORIES

One great feature of Mr. Alexander's system as seen in practical use is that the individual loses every suggestion of strain. He becomes perfectly 'lissom' in body; all strains and tensions disappear, and his body works like an oiled machine. Moreover, his system has a reflex result upon the mind of the patient, and a general condition of buoyancy and freedom, and indeed of gaiety of spirit takes the place of the old jaded mental position. It is the pouring in of new wine, but the bottles must also be new or they will burst, and this is exactly what Mr. Alexander's treatment does. It creates the new bottles and then the new wine can be poured in, freely and fully.

REV. W. PENNYMAN MA

The best way to understand how people, from all walks of life, can be helped is to hear from them personally, so I asked several people from my evening classes to write a short summary about how the Alexander Technique had helped them. I have not changed in any way the words in which they expressed themselves.

THE CASE HISTORY WITH WHICH I AM MOST FAMILIAR IS MY OWN, SO I WILL START WITH MYSELF:

It all started one cold, dark evening in January. I was driving my car along an unlit street when all of a sudden the two inner wheels of the car had left the road and I travelled for quite a few yards at an angle of 45 degrees, after which I landed with a large bump. I had, in fact, driven over a two-foot high pile of scaffold boards, which had been hidden in the darkness.

After a few days I started to develop backache so acute that I could hardly move. After a month or two the backache had eased, leaving me with sciatica. I went to my doctor who gave me some pain-killers and told me to rest. After being off work for six weeks the pain was no better, if anything it was worse. I was then put on a waiting list to see the back specialist at the local hospital. After many X-rays and various examinations no one was any the wiser as to why I still had the pain.

Nearly a year had elapsed. I was then referred to another specialist, but to no avail. All this time the sciatica remained. After another six months I was asked to attend the physiotherapy department for treatment; this did bring some relief, but only for a matter of hours. At this point I was offered a choice; either I would have to undergo a major operation, knowing that the surgeon did not know what was wrong, or I could go into a residential physiotherapy hospital. After a week of intensive treatment my back was hurting more than ever, so I discharged myself without any hope of a cure.

After a short while I started to see an osteopath, which really helped to relieve the pain, but again only temporarily. He did, however, suggest I try the Alexander Technique.

I had heard of it by name, but never quite knew what it was. Within a short period of time I had learnt how to help myself; the pain gradually began to ease, a great relief after nearly three years of constant discomfort. Within a month of starting my lessons I was able to stop taking the pain-killers that had become part and parcel of my life.

My mental and emotional states also improved, because there is nothing like continuous pain to make one feel depressed and worn out.

PATSY SPIERS. AGE: 49. OCCUPATION: MIDWIFE.

Patsy started coming to a day class with twelve others. She was suffering from a stiff neck that gave her pain whenever she turned her head. She was also prone to frequent and severe migraine headaches, and she had a wheezy chest which had led to her first asthma attack and greatly worried her.

After attending the class for two terms, including a little individual work, she reported:

The Alexander Technique, which is a way of allowing the body and mind to work together in order to avoid muscular tension, has constantly helped me to be calmer in stressful situations. It has also aided me to be more relaxed whilst driving. The stiff and painful neck has returned to normal, my wheeziness has improved greatly with no sign of the asthma returning, and my migraines are far less frequent and not nearly so intense. Although I feel I have a long way to go, I'm a lot more aware of myself, so whenever I get twinges of pain I adjust accordingly and the pain immediately eases. Although I still suffer from headaches, it takes a lot more physical and mental stress before it manifests.

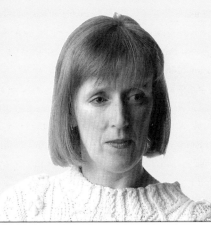

PAT VINCE. AGE: 58.
OCCUPATION: BANK CLERK.

When Pat came to me she was suffering from osteoarthritis of the neck and spine, and had raised blood pressure. She had tried everything, including osteopaths, chiropractors, physiotherapy, traction and pain-killers. She had this to say about her experience of the Technique:

I knew absolutely nothing about the Alexander Technique and viewed it with a certain amount of scepticism. I did not hope for very much when I began my lessons, because of past experiences. My main aim was for some relief to the back pain that I had had for many years but I was not too optimistic. I was also interested in the possible help for tension, worry and high blood pressure.

Now nearly a year later, attending one class a week and one weekend workshop, and no private lessons, I have been transformed by the Technique. I have found great relief from back pain, my tension and worry is very much reduced, and my doctor has given up even taking my blood pressure.

I have become much more aware of the workings of my body and have begun to use it in a way that is much more economical. I become aware when parts of my body become tense and I know now how to 'relax' them, and when my body is saying that it has had enough I am able to leave things till tomorrow instead of insisting that they have to be done today. The lessons on the causes and remedies of worry were most beneficial and the psychology of using your mind in order to create a change in the body helped to reduce the constant tensions in my mind, with the result that I am a much less tense person and a lot of my worries have just vanished.

I realize that I have much more to learn, but I am more than happy with the benefits that I have received so far.

PATRICK STANTON. AGE: 35.
OCCUPATION: BUILDER.

Patrick had fallen off a ladder over a year and a half ago and had been off work for much of that time. Although his initial injury had healed in a short time, he had been left with a pain in his left knee; this was made worse whenever he put pressure on the joint.

After having only ten weekly lessons he had this to say:

I had been in constant pain, since my accident, for nearly two years when I stumbled across the Alexander Technique. I had become withdrawn and at times very depressed, which, of course, had repercussions on my family. They were very sympathetic, but after a while the tension began to build, with ever-increasing rows.

I couldn't go back to work although I had tried several times and socializing was no fun at all. The pain and torment were beginning to take over my life.

After my fourth or fifth lesson I was able to see that it was I who was causing myself the discomfort. I had got into the habit of tensing up my left leg, which I probably did, initially, when I had my accident. I couldn't believe it at first that the problem was so simple; in fact I walked out of that lesson without any pain at all the first time for twenty months. The pain did, in fact, return the next day, but this experience had given me hope so I persevered with the lessons and now I am free of the pain for at least 95 per cent of the time. During the process, however, I have learnt so much about myself that I would never have known otherwise. I am deeply grateful to the Technique and to my teacher for the patience that he had.

VAL OATLEY. AGE: 62.
OCCUPATION: FORMER BALLET DANCER.

When Val came to me, in October 1989, she had arthritis in both her hands and feet, her shoulders and neck were in pain and she also suffered from chronic sciatica. After completing a course of day classes she had this to say:

By means of the Alexander Technique I have acquired an awareness of where my body is in space, which means I am now able to control my muscle tension by means of my brain; this is essential if I was ever to maintain a posture without straining my body unconsciously.

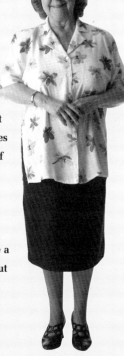

I have discovered a completeness of my mind and body so that it can work as a whole entity, instead of as a jumble of separate limbs, head and torso all working independently of one another. This, of course, relieves a lot of unnecessary muscle tension and teaches me a way of restoring the completeness of the body in a relaxed and coordinated way that had been lost in my early childhood.

Most of my aches and pains have dropped away leaving me able to achieve a balance and poise not only of the body, but of the mind as well.

49

Yvonne Dartnall. Age: 49.
Occupation: Owns and Runs a Hotel.

When Yvonne joined my classes she was suffering from tense shoulders and migraines that were very frequent and so intense that all she could do during an attack was lie down. After attending a regular two-hour class for seven months she wrote:

In my late forties, I was reaching a very difficult period of my life, for no matter what the ailment I was informed by my doctor and friends, 'Don't worry – it's just your age dear. You will just have to put up with it.' I found this difficult to believe but, before I continue, I will tell you a little about myself. When I was forty I suffered from my very first migraine, I was in bed for five days with it. Before this point in my life I had never really been ill.

The attacks became more and more frequent, with three or four each year and, by the time I had reached the age of 48 they were a fortnightly affair and almost unbearable. Any visit to the doctor always resulted in a prescribed medication that was ineffective.

I tried an osteopath and was able to get a little relief from minor repositioning of the discs, but I was becoming so tense that my head, neck and even my eyes were always painful. It was then that I decided to go along to the local college and enrol in what appeared to me to be 'a way to relax' – the Alexander Technique.

That was seven months ago.

My last migraine of any consequence was over four months ago, but I would not be so brash as to say that I have been cured. I can now take precautionary action, however, to limit the severity of the attack and even sometimes prevent the attack itself.

Hopefully, in the near future, I will say that I am cured, but I do know that whatever I have learned through the Alexander Technique, will help me through any other crisis in the future.

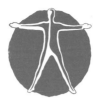

HOW DOES THE ALEXANDER TECHNIQUE WORK?

CHAPTER FOUR

'My technique is based on inhibition, the inhibition of undesirable, unwanted responses to stimuli, and hence it is primarily a technique for the development of the control of human reaction.'

FREDERICK MATTHIAS ALEXANDER

The Alexander Technique is a way of becoming more aware of both body and mind. It is based upon two main principles: 1. Inhibition 2. Direction.

By applying these two principles you will quickly see how unaware so many of us are as we go about our day-to-day lives.

We are nature's unique experiment to make the rational intelligence prove sounder than the reflex. Success or failure of this experiment depends on the basic human ability to impose a delay between the stimulus and the response.

JACOB BRONOWSKI

INHIBITION

Alexander defined inhibition as stopping yourself doing something that is a habit. He realized that, in order to bring about the changes he was seeking, he would first have to inhibit (or stop) the way that he was used to reacting in certain situations. By checking ourselves a moment before taking action, we give ourselves time to think about the most efficient and appropriate way of carrying out that action. This is a vital step towards having the power to choose freely on every level.

In this way, we see that before the brain is used for ACTION, it first can be used for INACTION. The ability to DELAY (pause) our responses until we are properly prepared is what is meant by INHIBITION. This moment of pausing before acting has nothing to do with freezing or performing actions slowly.

INSTINCTIVE INHIBITION

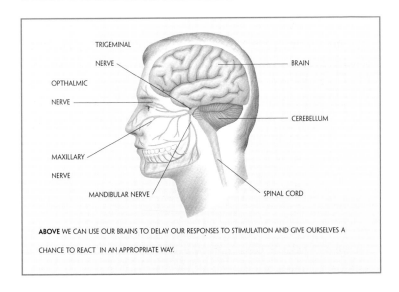

TRIGEMINAL NERVE

BRAIN

OPTHALMIC NERVE

CEREBELLUM

MAXILLARY NERVE

MANDIBULAR NERVE

SPINAL CORD

ABOVE WE CAN USE OUR BRAINS TO DELAY OUR RESPONSES TO STIMULATION AND GIVE OURSELVES A CHANCE TO REACT IN AN APPROPRIATE WAY.

The best examples of natural and instinctive inhibition are shown in the cat family. Even the domestic cat, when it first sees a mouse, does not immediately rush to capture its prey; instead, it waits until the right moment, when it is most likely to be successful.

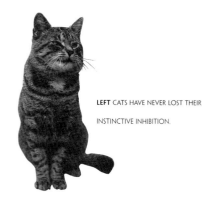

LEFT CATS HAVE NEVER LOST THEIR INSTINCTIVE INHIBITION.

'A cat inhibits the desire to spring prematurely and controls to a deliberate end its eagerness for the instant gratification of a natural appetite.'

FREDERICK MATTHIAS ALEXANDER

It is an interesting fact that, while being fine examples of inhibition and control, cats are also amongst the fastest creatures on earth.

53

The cat's ability to pause is part of its instinct – in other words, the cat does not think about doing it. Man, by contrast, can control his ability to pause, and it is this very difference that clearly divides him from the animal world.

Alexander firmly believed that man has to delay his immediate response to the many things that happen to him each day if he is ever to cope with his rapidly changing environment. As man has become less dependent on his body in order to survive, his instinct has become increasingly unreliable. Man must therefore use his mind to make up for this unreliability.

CONSCIOUS INHIBITION

If we are ever to change the way we react to things that happen to us we have to make a conscious decision to refuse to act in old automatic and unconscious patterns; that is, to say 'no' to our habits.

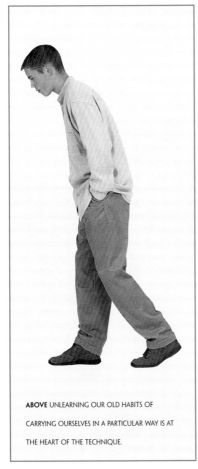

ABOVE UNLEARNING OUR OLD HABITS OF CARRYING OURSELVES IN A PARTICULAR WAY IS AT THE HEART OF THE TECHNIQUE.

By inhibiting our habits we have the choice to make different decisions. Inhibition is an essential step in practising the Technique.

Alexander described it in this way:

'Boiled down, it all comes to inhibiting a particular reaction to a given stimulus – but no one will see it that way. They will see it as getting in and out of a chair the right way. It is nothing of the kind. It is that a pupil decides what he will, or will not, consent to do.'

If you can stop yourself performing actions that put undue strain on your body then you are already halfway to your goal. Not performing an action is as much an act as actually performing it because, in both cases, the nervous system is used.

There are many ways of practising inhibition in daily life. For example, every time the telephone or doorbell rings, pause for two seconds before answering (you may find this simple exercise harder than it might seem!); or, if you find yourself in a heated discussion or argument, count backwards from ten to one before speaking. (This useful exercise in inhibition will give you time to think about what you really want to say.)

Try placing a chair in front of a mirror. Stand up and sit down in your normal way and see if you can notice any habits (anything that happens every time). Do not worry if you cannot see these straightaway. Then repeat the above but, this time, pause for a moment before any action while you consciously refuse to sit down or stand up in your normal way. Soon you will realize that there are many different ways of doing the same action. Can you notice any differences between the first and second ways of performing this action?

You may need to carry out the above exercises a few times before you start to become more aware of your actions.

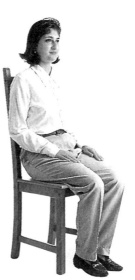

55

RIGHT YOU CAN LEARN A GREAT DEAL BY WATCHING YOURSELF IN A MIRROR AS YOU PERFORM A FAMILIAR ACTION, SUCH AS SITTING DOWN.

THE PRIMARY CONTROL

One of the most noticeable tendencies that Alexander observed in himself was the constant tightening of his neck muscles. At first, he presumed that this was just a personal habit, but he later found that nearly everybody tenses up their neck muscles. The habit usually leads to a pulling back of the head onto the spine, thus squeezing together the discs and shortening the structure of the body. This constant pressure on the spine is the main reason for people 'shrinking' with age.

The pulling back of the head also interferes dramatically with what Alexander called the 'Primary Control' (the relationship between the head, neck and back, which acts as the body's main organizer). Primary Control affects all the other reflexes and muscles throughout the body.

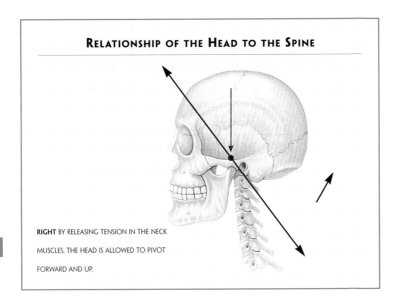

RELATIONSHIP OF THE HEAD TO THE SPINE

RIGHT BY RELEASING TENSION IN THE NECK MUSCLES, THE HEAD IS ALLOWED TO PIVOT FORWARD AND UP.

EXPERIMENTAL EVIDENCE

A professor of pharmacology, Rudolph Magnus, was very interested in exploring the role that physical movements play in affecting mental and emotional well-being. Magnus performed many experiments to find how the body holds its posture, and found that the head-neck reflex was the central controlling mechanism of an animal. It helps to put an animal into the correct position for a particular action and also helps to restore the animal to rest after an action.

Magnus' experiments, which took place around 1925, only confirmed what Alexander had discovered in himself a quarter of a century earlier: that all animals' body mechanisms are set up in such a way that the head leads a movement and the body then follows. This occurs naturally in all animals except for man whose head is

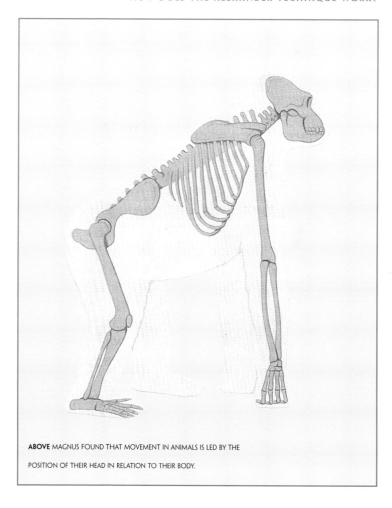

ABOVE MAGNUS FOUND THAT MOVEMENT IN ANIMALS IS LED BY THE
POSITION OF THEIR HEAD IN RELATION TO THEIR BODY.

frequently thrown back when a movement takes place.

A simple exercise can demonstrate this excess tension in the neck
muscles: sit in a chair and place either hand on the back of the neck
so that the two middle fingers just meet in the middle of the neck at
the base of the skull. Stand up, then sit down again, focusing your
attention on your hands to detect any pulling back of the head. If you
repeat this a few times, you may well notice more tension on the
second or third occasion.

IMPLICATIONS OF INTERFERING WITH THE PRIMARY CONTROL

If we are in the habit of pulling back our heads, and interfering with the Primary Control, then the implications are very serious indeed. Coordination and balance will be severely affected so much so that we hold ourselves rigid in order to avoid falling over. When we come to move we may actually be working against ourselves.

A clear example of this may be seen in the learner driver who grips the steering wheel so tightly with one hand that he has great difficulty in moving the wheel with the other. As a driving instructor I encountered many people who thought that there was something wrong with the car because the wheel would not move easily.

The interference with Primary Control builds up gradually, over a period of many years, and because of this most of us are unaware that we move in inefficient, and in many cases harmful, ways. Even when our bodies give us very clear signals that something is wrong, we rarely realize that we are causing the problem ourselves.

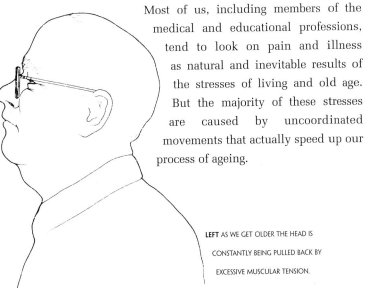

Most of us, including members of the medical and educational professions, tend to look on pain and illness as natural and inevitable results of the stresses of living and old age. But the majority of these stresses are caused by uncoordinated movements that actually speed up our process of ageing.

LEFT AS WE GET OLDER THE HEAD IS CONSTANTLY BEING PULLED BACK BY EXCESSIVE MUSCULAR TENSION.

The other major discovery that Magnus made he called the 'righting reflex'. He noticed that, after an action requiring extra tension (a cat leaping onto a table, for example), a set of 'righting reflexes' comes into play, returning the body to its normal posture.

The relationship of the head, neck and back is an essential part of returning our bodies to the right position. Therefore, when a person stiffens their neck muscles and pulls back their head, not only are they stopping their body being naturally coordinated, but they are preventing their body from returning to its natural state of ease.

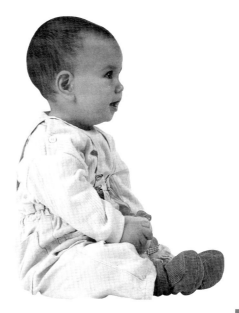

ABOVE INFANTS NATURALLY HOLD THEIR HEAD, NECK AND BACK IN ALIGNMENT – AS ADULTS THIS IS THE STATE WE WANT TO RETURN TO.

59

The key to freeing the body and to regaining its lost dignity lies in inhibiting the unconscious habit of muscle tension; only then may we perform actions in such a way that they become a joy to carry out.

SUMMARY

'What a piece of work is a man! How noble in reason! How infinite in faculty! In form and moving how express and admirable! In action how like an angel! In apprehension how like a god! The beauty of the world! The paragon of animals!'

Alexander found himself at odds with these famous words of Shakespeare:

'What could be less noble in reason, less infinite in faculty, than that man, despite his potentialities, should have fallen into such error in the use of himself, and in this way brought about such a lowering in his standard of functioning that in everything he attempts to accomplish, these harmful conditions tend to become more and more exaggerated. In consequence, how many people are there today of whom it may be said, as regards their use of themselves, "in form and moving how express and admirable"?'

In his own personal development, Alexander became convinced that if he was able to stop doing the 'wrong' thing, then the 'right' thing would automatically happen. But first he had to inhibit his habitual responses. For most of us, the habit of acting without thinking about it first is very deeply ingrained and, therefore, is not an easy one to 'break'. Neither do we realize how important it is to inhibit our automatic responses.

Many people think that inhibition means suppressing their natural responses. This is not correct. Inhibition does not mean that you have to stop being spontaneous.

DIRECTION

'You come to learn to inhibit and to direct your activity. You learn, first, to inhibit the habitual reaction to certain classes of stimuli, and, second, to direct yourself consciously in such a way as to affect certain muscular pulls, which processes bring about a new reaction to these stimuli.'

F.M. ALEXANDER

As part of his experimentation, Alexander asked himself what he had been looking to for direction in his actions. He realized that he had been relying on a sense of what seemed 'natural' and 'right'. As his research had proved these feelings to be unreliable, he therefore decided to put together instructions to himself to replace them.

To give directions is to project messages from the brain to the body and then to give energy to the body to carry out the directions.

You can direct specific parts of the body – for example, you can think of your fingers lengthening – and you can direct your whole body – by thinking of your whole structure lengthening. You can also direct your body to move by consciously deciding where you are going to, and letting the head lead the movement while the rest of your body follows.

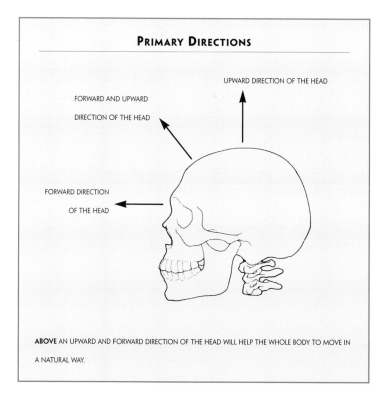

PRIMARY DIRECTIONS

UPWARD DIRECTION OF THE HEAD

FORWARD AND UPWARD
DIRECTION OF THE HEAD

FORWARD DIRECTION
OF THE HEAD

ABOVE AN UPWARD AND FORWARD DIRECTION OF THE HEAD WILL HELP THE WHOLE BODY TO MOVE IN
A NATURAL WAY.

MAIN DIRECTIONS

Alexander realized that the root cause of many problems was the over-tightening of the neck muscles, causing an interference with the Primary Control and so throwing the whole body out of balance. The first and most important step, therefore, was to give the orders to ensure a lessening of tension in the neck area so that the Primary Control could be allowed to work properly again.

The directions he devised were as follows:

1. **Allow the neck to be free so that**

2. **the head can go forward and upwards in order that**

3. **the back can lengthen and widen.**

ALLOW THE NECK TO BE FREE

This instruction is needed to get rid of excessive tension in the muscles of the neck. This is essential if the head is to be free in relation to the rest of the body, so that the Primary Control can work properly. This direction should always be given first because other directions will not work without it.

ALLOW THE HEAD TO GO FORWARDS AND UPWARDS

The head is balanced in such a way that, when the neck muscles are released, the head goes slightly forward, taking the whole body into movement. This direction, therefore, helps the body to perform its natural functions. If one thought of the head only going forward, and not upward, it would usually drop downwards, causing more tension in the neck muscles. It is important to realize that the head should go forward in relation to the spine. The upward direction of the head is away from the spine and not away from the earth (although these may be the same when the structure is upright),

ALLOW THE BACK TO LENGTHEN AND WIDEN

Since the spine shortens when muscular tension pulls the head back, it follows that by allowing the head to release forward and up, the whole body will lengthen. Many people who practise the Alexander Technique increase in height by an inch or more. The widening direction is necessary because it is very easy for a narrowing to occur at the same time as lengthening.

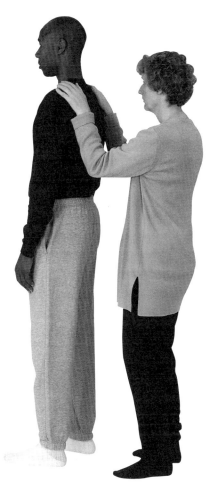

ABOVE A TRAINED ALEXANDER TECHNIQUE TEACHER CAN HELP YOU TO GIVE THE DIRECTIONS ACCURATELY.

These three primary directions are, in themselves, very simple and straightforward. They can be quite confusing however, partly because we find it difficult to accept that the solution to a long-standing problem could be so simple; confusion may also arise because we presume that we are doing something wrong when we do not achieve immediate results. The answer to this is to be patient and realize that you are changing the habits of a lifetime.

It is strongly advisable that, before you start to give directions, you have at least a few lessons from a trained Alexander teacher to make sure you are on the right track, as this could save you a great deal of time and trouble. (A list of contact numbers for finding a teacher can be found in the back of this book.)

SECONDARY DIRECTIONS

There are many secondary directions, too numerous to mention here. Whereas the primary directions can be applied to everyone, the secondary may be applied to certain conditions or ailments. For example, if a person came to me suffering from rounded shoulders I might give him or her an instruction to 'think of your shoulders releasing away from each other'. Or, if someone came to me with arthritis of the fingers, I might ask him to 'think of your fingers lengthening'.

Some examples of secondary directions commonly used in the teaching of the Technique are given on the following pages.

There are many more directions that can be given, according to the individual, but the primary directions should always come before any secondary direction. The word 'allow' may often be substituted for the words 'think of' – try both and note the different effects on the body. The most important factor to remember is to 'think' or 'allow'. Never try to DO anything as this will always increase muscular tension, which is the very opposite of what you are trying to achieve.

WHEN SITTING

- Think of the shoulders going away from each other (for rounded shoulders).

- Think of the sitting bones releasing into the chair (for arched back).

- Think of the feet lengthening and widening (for collapsed arches).

- Think of the shoulders dropping away from ears (for hunched shoulders).

- Think of the elbows dropping away from shoulders (for tension in the arms and shoulders).

- Think of the hands lengthening and widening (for tense hands).

- Think about not arching the back (for arched back).

- Think of the ribcage dropping downwards (for breathing problems).

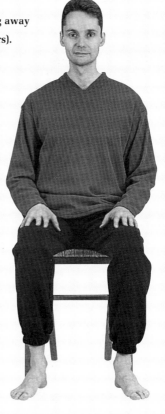

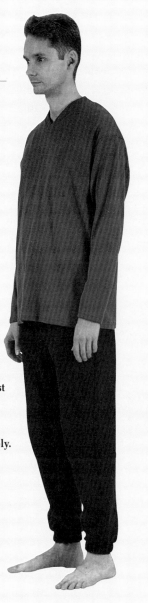

WHEN STANDING MOST OF THE DIRECTIONS FROM SITTING APPLY AS WELL AS THE FOLLOWING:

- Think of a lengthening between feet and head (general).

- Think of letting your weight go evenly through the soles of your feet (for balance).

- Think of not bracing the knees back (for excess tension in the legs).

- Think of not pushing the hips forward (for backache).

- Think of lengthening between the navel and the upper part of the chest (for depression).

When walking many of the above apply.

RIGHT DIRECTION

The last type of direction is that of directing your body as a whole – 'What is the direction that I am going in?'

Many people associate the Alexander Technique with putting particular parts of the body into certain positions that they then hold in place, thinking that this is improved posture. But holding these positions only creates extra muscular tension, replacing one habit with another. The Technique sets out to do precisely the opposite of this: parts of the body remain free from other parts no matter what position you may adopt. This, of course, is essential for free movement to take place.

Alexander was adamant that there was no such thing as a right position, but there was such a thing as a right direction. In other words, there's no correct way of sitting, standing or moving but there should be a lengthening of the body during these exercises.

Directions, along with inhibition, form the backbone of the Alexander Technique. By applying these two principles, you will be able to change your old habitual ways of moving and will, in turn, experience a new and improved use of yourself. Consequently, you will slowly be able to eliminate many ailments that have been caused by long-standing patterns of misuse.

'Yesterday is but a cancelled check
Tomorrow is an I.O.U
Today is the only hard cash you possess…
Spend it wisely!'
ANON

'We do not see things as they are.
We see them as we are.'
THE TALMUD

CONSCIOUSNESS

The key to learning the Technique is awareness. At first, to be aware of how we perform various activities seems very alien, because we are used to moving automatically without any thought whatsoever. Slowly we are taught to think briefly before performing any given action and then to be aware of muscle tension as we perform different actions.

Most people are surprised when they find out that they are causing their neck or back muscles to tense needlessly. By analysing even simple movements, such as walking, bending or getting up from a chair, we can find new ways of moving that help us to release tension rather than create it. People who have undergone a course of lessons often experience less tiredness and have more energy to do the things they enjoy, instead of sitting around each evening feeling exhausted. In this way the quality of their lives is greatly enhanced and feelings of calmness, happiness and a greater sense of well-being are often reported.

It is very rare that we give much attention to ourselves apart from our appearance - we may well spend a lot of money on clothes, make-up and perfume in trying to look attractive and yet there is nothing more beautiful than someone who is moving gracefully or standing with poise.

Many people who have taken lessons say that the Technique has helped them to look and feel years younger, which is something nearly everyone would like to achieve! In addition, it will not only help you to be more aware of your body, but also of the world about you. You will have a greater appreciation of life in general, as many worries and concerns begin to fade.

'If we are truly in the present moment, and are not being carried away by our thoughts and fantasies, then we are in a position to be free of fate and available to our destiny. When we are in the present moment, our work on Earth begins.'

RESHAD FIELD

'Use your eyes as if tomorrow you would be stricken blind. And the same method can be applied to other senses. Hear the music of voices, the song of the birds, the mighty strains of an orchestra, as if you would be stricken deaf tomorrow. Touch each object you want to touch as if tomorrow your tactile sense would fail. Smell the perfume of flowers, taste with relish each morsel, as if tomorrow you could never smell and taste again.

Make the most of every sense.'

HELEN KELLER

RE-EDUCATION

When you begin to apply the principles of the Technique you will not be learning anything new, but simply unlearning many habits that you have acquired during the course of your life. Frederick Matthias Alexander, the originator of the Technique, said often that if you stopped doing the wrong thing (i.e. the habit) the right thing would happen by itself. It is, however, sometimes harder to relearn it than it is to learn something in the first place, because our normal way of performing actions feels so right, but as you start to allow tension to release you will find that you are naturally using your body in a much more balanced and co-ordinated way. Any aches or pain will slowly ease, and eventually disappear altogether.

'There's only one corner of the universe you can be certain of improving and that's your own self.'
ALDOUS HUXLEY

'Alexander established not only the beginnings of a far reaching science of the apparently involuntary movements we call reflexes, but a technique of correction and self control which forms a substantial addition to our very slender resources in personal education.'
GEORGE BERNARD SHAW

> It is important to realise that the whole process of re-evaluating the way in which you move does take time, as you are dealing with habits that have been present since childhood. As the pace of life increases it seems that we often expect results immediately, and yet nature is not like that. It will take time for the body to restructure itself and it may even take a few lessons just to comprehend what is being asked of you.

CHANGING YOUR PATTERNS OF BEHAVIOUR

Throughout our lives we all develop physical, mental and emotional patterns of behaviour and it is often the case that other people are more aware of them than we are. We react to a given situation over and over again in a set way, irrespective of whether or not it is appropriate, and as many of these reactions are unconscious, we will repeat them time after time without being aware of it. Most of these ways of responding were learnt as a child and some of them started even before our earliest childhood memory.

As I have mentioned before, a good example of habitual behaviour arises when we are running late for work or an appointment. It is easy to see the reaction of someone who is stressed by time, by their hunched shoulders, their arched back and their head going back. They no longer think rationally, and when driving may take unnecessary risks as they fear the consequences of being late, sometimes even when the appointment is of little importance, such as meeting a friend for a drink. We may even risk our lives in this stressed state. It is important to realise that 'life is not an emergency' so take your time. This old proverb might help:

> **There is never the time to do a job properly,**
> **But there is always time to come back and correct the mistakes.**

'Between stimulus and response, there is a space.
In that space lies our freedom and power to choose
our response. In our response lies our growth
and our happiness.'

ANON

'We learn wisdom from failure much more
than from success;
we often discover what will do, by finding
out what will not do;
and probably he who never made a mistake
never made a discovery.'

SAMUEL SMILES

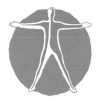

HELPING YOURSELF

CHAPTER FIVE

'By and through consciousness and the application
of a reasoning intelligence, man may rise above the
powers of all disease and physical disabilities.
This triumph is not to be won in sleep, in trance,
in submission, in paralysis, or in anaesthesia,
but in a clear, open-eyed, reasoning, deliberate
consciousness by mankind.'

FREDERICK MATTHIAS ALEXANDER

The first question that everyone asks, when in pain, is 'What can I do to help myself?' But really this is the wrong question because most of us are doing far too much already. Maybe the question, 'What is it that I have to undo in order to help myself?' is more appropriate when it comes to the Alexander Technique. In order to answer this we first have to become aware of ourselves and how we go about certain actions.

We are all taught from a very early age that if we are going to get anywhere in this life, we have got to make effort. To a point this may be true, but often that effort results in over-exerting ourselves, and leaving us exhausted. We are then robbed of the improved quality of life that we are aiming for. Alexander referred to this behaviour as 'end-gaining'.

At first, being so aware of ourselves may seem very strange; this is because we are not used to it. Even when we do become more aware, how do we know whether what we are doing is 'right' or 'wrong'? Well, no one movement can be said to be wrong, it is the repetition of a movement that begins to put a strain upon the body. So the more aware we are, the less likely it is that the way we carry out our activities will become habitual.

Look at children while they are walking. Sometimes they will walk fast, even running from place to place, and then they will skip or hop, and the next moment they may be walking quite slowly (much to their mothers' annoyance). The size of their steps is also very varied. Yet you can often recognize an adult by the way he or she walks. This is because our movements slowly become stereotyped as life goes on and we tend to move in a way that feels 'right' to us. We never question that feeling, we just go on in our habitual ways until we are stopped short by illnesses. Even then, we rarely realize that many of these ailments are, directly or indirectly, brought about by the way in which we think and move.

Alexander said that everyone wants to be right but no one stops to think whether their idea of right is in fact right. He called this very common human condition 'faulty sensory perception'.

73

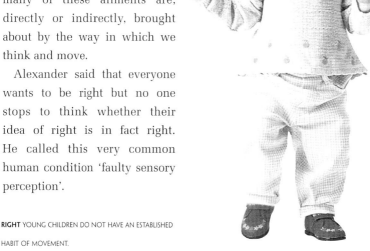

RIGHT YOUNG CHILDREN DO NOT HAVE AN ESTABLISHED HABIT OF MOVEMENT.

UNRELIABLE SENSORY FEELINGS

The main problem that people come across as they begin to practise the Alexander Technique is the same as Alexander experienced when he was developing his Technique, that is, an 'unreliable sensory feedback mechanism'. In other words, the actions that we intend to do may be completely different from those that we actually carry out.

As you will remember, Alexander discovered that the cause of his vocal problem was that he was pulling his head back and down onto his spine. Until he saw this in the mirror, he had been completely unaware of it. His sensory feedback had not informed him that this was happening even though the tension needed to throw his head back had been tremendous.

Even when he tried to put this matter right, by putting his head forward and up, he was faced with an even greater difficulty because he saw again from the mirror that he was increasing the tension and pulling his head back even further. He could hardly believe his eyes and it was then he knew that he was unable to rely on his sensory feelings. Everyone I have ever taught is also a victim of faulty sensory perception in one form or another.

If most of us cannot tell where our body is in space, then it follows that we may be walking, sitting, standing or moving in a way that is putting enormous stresses on ourselves without realizing it. The body is by nature very resilient, and it may only be years later that the effects of this misuse become apparent to us. It is true to say that in many cases the seeds of future ill health are already sown by the age of fifteen or sixteen. When applying the Technique, one of the first lessons we need to learn is that our sensory feelings are faulty; only then is it possible to start making the changes necessary to relieve the muscular tension that lies at the heart of the pattern of the misuse of ourselves. Faulty sensory perception is one of the hardest obstacles to overcome when learning the Alexander Technique, and this is the main reason why it is essential for you to find a teacher who can guide you safely through a maze of these unreliable feelings.

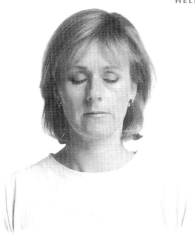

ABOVE WITH OUR EYES CLOSED, MOST OF US MISJUDGE WHAT WE ARE DOING WITH OUR BODIES.

As an example of unreliable sensory feeling try closing your eyes and, using your senses and feelings only, place your feet so that they are twelve inches (0.3 metre) apart, parallel with each other.

Now open your eyes and see whether the feet are, indeed, parallel and if they are a foot apart. Most people will see that what they feel and what actually happens are two totally different things. Now, with your eyes open, place your feet parallel – many people will feel that their feet are pointing inwards.

Remember that this is not the correct way to stand, it is just an exercise to demonstrate that we cannot rely upon our feelings to tell us about what we are doing to ourselves. Faulty sensory appreciation does not just relate to our feet, but to the whole of the rest of our body.

In all his years of teaching, Alexander did not come across anyone who did not experience the same problem. So you can see that, without professional help, we can make our problems worse, even with the best of intentions.

AWARENESS

The only thing we can do to help ourselves is to become more aware of how we go about simple actions. This will help to bring our minds back into the present more often. Even just being more conscious will help you to perform many actions with greater ease and efficiency of movement.

If you notice a particular position that causes discomfort or pain, such as sitting or standing for long periods, do as Alexander did and use a mirror to help you discover the source of your problem.

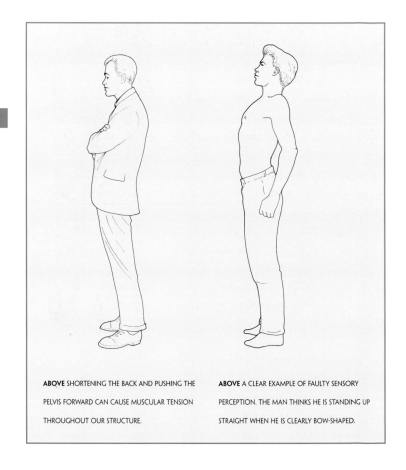

ABOVE SHORTENING THE BACK AND PUSHING THE PELVIS FORWARD CAN CAUSE MUSCULAR TENSION THROUGHOUT OUR STRUCTURE.

ABOVE A CLEAR EXAMPLE OF FAULTY SENSORY PERCEPTION. THE MAN THINKS HE IS STANDING UP STRAIGHT WHEN HE IS CLEARLY BOW-SHAPED.

As you can see from the figure on the previous page the man thinks that he is standing up straight when anyone can see that he is leaning backwards from the waist. This, if allowed to continue, would cause chronic back pain in later life. Any one of us could be under the same sort of misapprehension without realizing it.

At first any new way of being is bound to feel strange, even unnatural, because we have become so used to moving in habitual ways. This strangeness will very quickly pass in the same way as a capped tooth or new filling feels peculiar after a visit to the dentist yet, after a couple of days, we do not even notice it any more.

In the same way, when a teacher adjusts you into an upright position you will probably feel as though you are falling forwards. This feeling will soon pass, however, and you will be left with a sense of poise and balance that had been long forgotten.

After having some Alexander lessons, you will begin to understand the principles of 'inhibition' and 'direction'. Soon you will find that you are taking more time to act, instead of reacting in an habitual way.

If there is one thing that really will make a difference to your life, it will be applying inhibition before carrying out any actions. At first it may not be easy… we will usually find that we

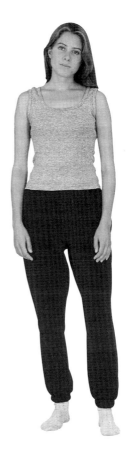

ABOVE WE HAVE ALL DEVELOPED HABITUAL WAYS OF HOLDING OURSELVES. THIS PERSON IS UNCONSCIOUSLY HOLDING HER HEAD TO THE LEFT.

77

have completed the task at hand and then we remember that we have not stopped to think first. Do not worry as this will get easier with practice.

You could start from today. Next time the phone rings or there is a knock on the door, just pause for a moment instead of reacting immediately. You may find that the level of stress in your body will very soon go down, especially if you are one of those millions of people who rush around every day trying to beat deadline after deadline.

Many people will say that they do not have the time to pause before acting, but this is a false economy; if you do not pause then nature has its own ways of making you stop through pain or illness.

A question to ask yourself is this: 'What is more important, the job that I am doing or myself?' We sometimes lose all perspective of what really is important in this life. Alexander realized that the right thing to do would be the last thing that we would think of doing, if left to ourselves.

Try the following movements to increase your self-awareness and help yourself.

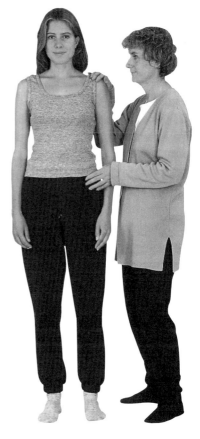

ABOVE WHEN AN ALEXANDER TECHNIQUE TEACHER POSITIONS YOU INTO A TRULY UPRIGHT POSITION, YOU WILL PROBABLY FEEL THAT YOU ARE LEANING TO THE RIGHT.

78

STANDING

If you have to stand for a while at work or in a queue, it would be helpful to have one leg behind the other with the feet at about 45 degrees to each other. The weight of the body should chiefly rest on the rear leg. In this way the hips cannot be pushed forward and therefore are able to support the torso more effectively, thus reducing any excess muscle strain. This will be especially helpful to those who suffer from lower back pain.

Be aware of your feet and where the body weight is being placed. Can you feel more weight on your toes or your heels? Is more weight thrown onto the inside or outside of each foot?

You can often answer these questions by closely examining an old pair of shoes to see the area of most wear.

There are three points of balance on the feet:

1. The heel.
2. The ball of the foot.
3. A point just below the big toe.

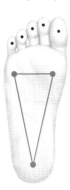

All three points should be in contact with the ground if we are to be truly stable. It is worth noting that we are in fact, 206 bones placed on top of one another, with the head, weighing approximately a stone, delicately balanced on the top. It is no wonder then that we have a tendency to be unstable.

Any photographer will tell you that a tripod is necessary in order for the camera on top to remain stable. In the same way all three points need to have equal weight going through them in order to maintain balance and coordination without placing an undue strain upon muscles and joints.

Having said that, it is important to point out that there is no one correct standing position.

SITTING

It is never a good idea to sit for long periods but, if this is essential, you should be sure to get up from time to time in order to move the body. If you do not do this the muscles may become fixed in a shortened state, putting a strain on joints and various internal organs.

The soles of the feet should be in contact with the ground because receptors in the feet directly activate the postural muscles throughout the torso. If these are not activated, by having the legs stretched out in front, for example, then you will end up sitting in a slumped manner. This will, of course, affect the breathing and other vital functions of the body.

There are also chairs that you can buy, designed by a chiropractor, that are intended to put less strain on the body when sitting. Full information about these chairs can be found on Page 115.

It might be useful at this point to discuss muscles. There are 650 muscles in the body; these contain two kinds of muscle fibres, which are known as voluntary and involuntary muscle fibres.

VOLUNTARY MUSCLES

The voluntary muscles are nearly always attached to the bones of the skeleton and their function is to move parts of the body when we wish them to.

They always work in pairs, one muscle shortening while its opposite lengthens, thus moving the bones to which they are attached. We can choose to make even the minutest of movements as and when we wish. These muscles can tire, however, after a short time.

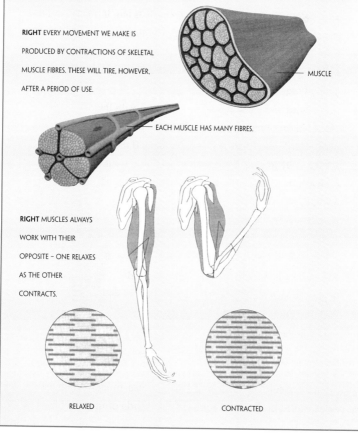

RIGHT EVERY MOVEMENT WE MAKE IS PRODUCED BY CONTRACTIONS OF SKELETAL MUSCLE FIBRES. THESE WILL TIRE, HOWEVER, AFTER A PERIOD OF USE.

MUSCLE

EACH MUSCLE HAS MANY FIBRES.

81

RIGHT MUSCLES ALWAYS WORK WITH THEIR OPPOSITE – ONE RELAXES AS THE OTHER CONTRACTS.

RELAXED

CONTRACTED

INVOLUNTARY MUSCLES

The involuntary muscles, on the other hand, cannot be used at will. They work when they are triggered by numerous reflexes situated throughout the body. These muscles have the function of keeping us upright against the ever-present force of gravity; they have the advantage of never tiring as they need to work for long periods at a time.

If the body is used in an uncoordinated fashion some of the reflexes are not being triggered. The muscles that control our posture are therefore not put to work. We then start to use our voluntary muscles for support – something for which they were not designed. As a result, we feel very tired after a comparatively short time.

The voluntary muscles are then contracted for long periods and, over the years, become shorter and shorter. This possibly, is one of the main reasons why, as people get older, they become shorter. People who have Alexander lessons, on the other hand, may gain height because the involuntary muscles start to work again and the other muscles become less tense and are allowed to lengthen.

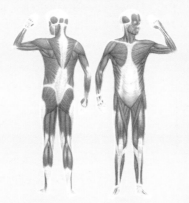

ABOVE OUR VOLUNTARY MUSCLES SHOULD NOT BE USED TO SUPPORT OUR BODY FOR LONG PERIODS – WHEN THEY ARE, THEY SOON BECOME TIRED.

WALKING

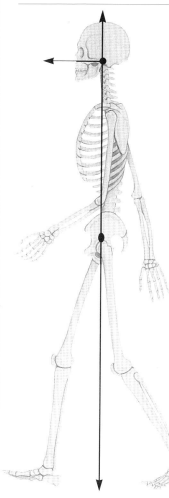

The main factor to remember about walking is to be aware of what is around you. It is easy to walk down the road and to be thinking of something else completely. Without us noticing, this will affect our whole balance and coordination. This is because 40 per cent of all the information that is taken in through the eyes is for balance alone. You can prove this for yourself: stand with one leg off the ground so that you are balanced on one leg, and then just close your eyes. Within a few moments you will start to lose your balance. So, if you are not aware of what is around you and are not purposeful in your movements you may be off balance. Your muscles are then required to work harder.

If you look at a small child's eyes, they are nearly always looking in the direction in which they are moving. Sadly, this is not the case with most adults.

83

ABOVE WHEN PERFECTLY ALIGNED, WE CAN MOVE THROUGH LIFE WITH GREATER EASE.

PICKING UP OBJECTS

Many people know that they should bend their knees when they bend down to pick up an object, but this is only half the story. The other half is that the hips have to bend also. This will keep the whole body in perfect balance and make the action of picking up an object into a simple activity. What so many people still do is bend from the waist while keeping their legs straight. The result is that they will be using their back muscles, instead of their huge thigh muscles, which are much better equipped to do the job. When you do not bend your knees then the back muscles have to support and pick up the weight of your torso, arms and head (about 70 per cent of your body weight), as well as the object you are carrying.

Many back injuries happen this way. The main reason why people act in this manner is to save a few seconds – a high price to pay.

It is interesting to watch professional weight lifters because they always use the thigh muscles to lift the very heavy weights – they have to.

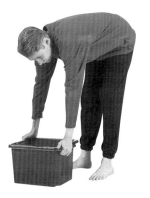 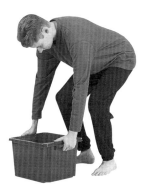

ABOVE BY BEING AWARE OF OUR MOVEMENTS WHEN LIFTING, WE CAN HELP PREVENT SERIOUS BACK PROBLEMS IN LATER LIFE.

SITTING DOWN

During this action we often misuse our body. If you look at people as they sit down, you can see for yourself that a great many of them fall backwards into their chairs. Whenever the body falls backwards a reflex in the neck (the fear reflex) is triggered: this causes the head to be pulled back onto the spine and the shoulders to be hunched. The reflex protects the very sensitive area at the bottom of the skull and, because it works by reflex, we cannot have conscious control over it. If it is stimulated every time we sit down then tremendous tensions will build up over the years; these will give rise to neck and back problems, and will also be responsible for many headaches and migraines. All you need to do to avoid this reflex is to bend your hips and knees so that your body is balanced until you reach the chair.

GETTING UP FROM A CHAIR

Most people use huge amounts of energy when performing this simple activity. This is because they try to get up before their body weight is over their feet. It is much easier to lean forward before attempting to rise or, if this is not possible, to bring the feet back so they are almost under the body.

When you have to get up from a settee, it will take less effort if you come to the edge of it before trying to stand.

Another common action is pushing down with the hands on to the legs to push the body upwards. This stops them from straightening, and the legs will then have to work a great deal harder in order to fight against your hands.

RIGHT BY ALLOWING THE HEAD TO LEAD WHEN STANDING UP FROM A CHAIR, WE WILL REDUCE THE EFFORT REQUIRED TO PERFORM THIS MOVEMENT.

LEANING FORWARD WHEN SITTING

This is a common activity that we all do when writing, typing and eating. To lean forward we usually shorten the front of the torso, which again will affect our breathing and all the internal organs. It is far better to lean forward from the hip joints, thus lengthening the whole body. Sitting on a forward sloping seat may help.

All these tips can be very useful in relieving some of the stress that we put on ourselves unknowingly. They are, however, just the tip of the iceberg. An understanding of how we are designed to move in this world is essential if we are to correct our bad habits, the source of much pain and discomfort. As we learn to give ourselves more time to pause before activity, we will slowly become more and more aware of the warning signals that our body gives us when it is under stress. In the past most of us have been unaware of these signs and that is why our body stops working normally. Our body is very strong and it is only after years and years of mistreatment that it finally says, 'I can't stand this any more.'

The idea of inhibition may seem easy to apply but, in my experience, this is not the case. It seems to go against our very nature. We have been taught from an early age to rush our activities and to be only interested in the end product. The way by which we reach that end is not valued, and yet our actions can be beautiful in themselves. Just look at a swan landing on water, a whale leaping out of the water, or a child playing on the beach – such beauty just in the movements.

RIGHT LEANING FORWARD IN THIS WAY WHILE SITTING SQUASHES THE INTERNAL ORGANS AND THEREFORE IMPAIRS THEIR PERFORMANCE.

BREATHING

The breath is the essence of life; breathing is the first thing you did when entering this world, and it will be the last thing you do when you leave. Everyone knows that breathing is the most fundamental requirement we have and without it we cannot survive for more than a few moments, yet most of us give it very little attention. In fact, our health and general well-being depend on the way we breathe and it is therefore vital that we relearn how to breathe naturally.

'People travel to wonder at the heights of mountains,
at the huge waves of the sea, at the long courses of rivers,
at the vast compass of the ocean, at the circular motion
of the stars; and they pass by themselves
without wondering'
SAINT AUGUSTINE

If you observe a baby or young child you will see that the abdomen moves in and out rhythmically with each breath, while the upper chest and shoulders remain in a state of relaxation and therefore relatively still. Yet in many adults the opposite happens; the abdomen remains rigid, forcing the ribcage to be pushed up on the in-breath and then to collapse on the out-breath. I find that when people first come for lessons, their breathing is often very erratic or too fast; they do not even give themselves time to finish one breath before they start the next. This is a direct reflection of how they are living their lives, and often they will say that they always feel that there are not enough hours in a day. The stress that many people are under causes excessive muscular tension, restricts the breathing and results in breathing habits which are detrimental to their bodily functions, their state of mind and their quality of life.

THE WHISPERED 'AH'

The first thing to do to improve your breathing is simply to become aware of the breath without trying to change it. Just by placing your attention on to how you breathe will bring about an improvement. Contrary to what many people think, it is the out-breath that controls the way we breathe, because it causes a vacuum in our lungs which allows the next inhalation to be taken spontaneously and without effort. To help his pupils relearn how to breath naturally, Alexander developed the following procedure, which is known as 'the whispered ah':

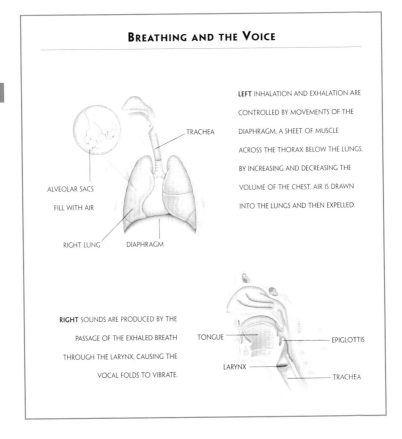

BREATHING AND THE VOICE

LEFT INHALATION AND EXHALATION ARE CONTROLLED BY MOVEMENTS OF THE DIAPHRAGM, A SHEET OF MUSCLE ACROSS THE THORAX BELOW THE LUNGS. BY INCREASING AND DECREASING THE VOLUME OF THE CHEST, AIR IS DRAWN INTO THE LUNGS AND THEN EXPELLED.

TRACHEA

ALVEOLAR SACS FILL WITH AIR

RIGHT LUNG   DIAPHRAGM

RIGHT SOUNDS ARE PRODUCED BY THE PASSAGE OF THE EXHALED BREATH THROUGH THE LARYNX, CAUSING THE VOCAL FOLDS TO VIBRATE.

TONGUE

LARYNX

EPIGLOTTIS

TRACHEA

THE WHISPERED 'AH' TECHNIQUE

First notice where your tongue is and let it rest with the tip lightly touching the lower front teeth.

1. Make sure your lips and facial muscles are not in tension.
   To assist this it may be helpful to think of something amusing.
2. After you finish your next in-breath, open your mouth by letting your jaw drop (make sure your head does not tilt backwards in the process).
3. Whisper an 'ah' sound until you come to the natural end of the breath.
4. Gently close your lips and allow the air to come in through your nose and fill up your lungs.
5. Repeat several times.

Regular practice of this technique will help you to notice detrimental breathing habits and will lead to a more efficient respiratory system. It is important to remain at peace when doing this exercise. In order to breathe more fully, it might be helpful to remember this quote:

'The same stream of life that runs through my veins night and day runs through the world and dances in rhythmic measures. It is the same life that shouts in joy through the dust of the Earth in numberless blades of grass and breaks into tumultuous waves of leaves and flowers. It is the same life that rocked in the ocean cradle of birth and of death, in ebb and in flow. I feel my limbs are made glorious by the touch of this world of life and my pride is from life throb of ages dancing in my blood this moment.'

RAHBINDRATH TAGORE

END-GAINING

This is a term that Alexander used to describe the nature of modern man. He blamed our 'end-gaining' nature for many of the problems that we face today.

A clear example can be seen in the case of the destruction of the rain forests, causing the greenhouse effect. For the sake of a handful of people making huge profits the entire planet has been put in danger.

In the same way we may stress ourselves at work, causing ulcers, backache and nervous breakdowns in the process, but for what? So that we can make money. Why do we want to make money? So that we can be happy. But when we have backaches, nervous problems or stress we are anything but happy. This way of thinking is not reasonable, yet we carry on in the same way, generation after generation, never learning by our past mistakes. What sets mankind apart from the rest of creation is intelligence, but we never stop long enough to put our intelligence to good use.

I once saw a cartoon that pictured hundreds of lemmings throwing themselves off a cliff and drowning in the water below. The caption below read:

'After all, 2000 lemmings can't be wrong.'

Yes, the Alexander Technique is a very useful tool that you can use to help you find the solutions to many physical, emotional and mental problems but, more than that, it has the potential to help us use our intelligence to help ourselves and our fellow man. Through technology we have advanced to a point where we can destroy this planet and everything on it. Now is the time to stop this end-gaining and think about what we really want in our lives.

'What lies behind us, and what lies before us are tiny matters, compared to what lies within us.'
RALPH WALDO EMERSON

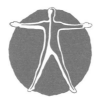

PRACTICAL EXERCISES

CHAPTER SIX

Although there are no exercises as such when practising the Alexander Technique, there are ways of relieving muscular tension in the body. The most common of these is lying on the floor with your head supported on books. The number of books does vary a great deal and your teacher will explain to you exactly how many books are required. If you want to do this for yourself the following method is not quite so accurate, but will give you the general idea.

BOOK SUPPORT

The number of books needed will depend upon your height and how curved your spine is. To find this out stand, as you would normally, with your heels, buttocks and shoulder blades lightly touching a wall. Get a friend to measure the distance between your head and the

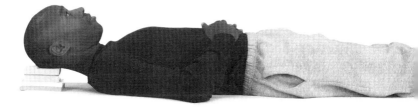

ABOVE THE HEIGHT OF THE PILE OF BOOKS POSITIONED UNDER THE HEAD IS CRUCIAL IN ENSURING THAT THE MOST BENEFIT IS REAPED FROM THIS EXERCISE.

wall and add about half an inch to the measurement. This will be the height of the books you will need. If you are still not sure, just remember that it is better to have too many books than too few. The number of books may vary as you slowly release the tension in the neck, so it is useful to recheck the number each month. Be sure that the books used are paperback as this will be more comfortable.

SEMI-SUPINE POSITION

Be aware of how you actually get down to the floor. Get onto all fours and gently roll onto the books. Your Alexander teacher will show you how to do this with the minimum of effort. As you are lying with the books under your head, bring your feet as near to your buttocks as is comfortably possible so that your knees are pointing to the ceiling. Have your hands gently resting either side of your navel.

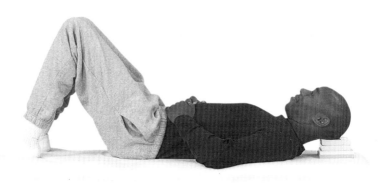

ABOVE WHILE LYING IN THIS POSITION, YOU SHOULD BECOME AWARE OF ANY MUSCLE TENSION IN ALL PARTS OF YOUR BOD – FEET, LEGS, BACK, SHOULDERS, ARMS AND HEAD.

Awareness While Lying

A good length of time to be in this position is about twenty minutes. While you are lying there try to become aware of any tensions in your body. You could ask yourself the following questions:

- Is my back arched so that it is not fully in contact with the ground?

- Are my shoulders hunched so that they are close to my ears?

- Are my shoulder blades not fully in contact with the ground because my shoulders tend to be rounded?

- Do the books feel very hard because I have a tendency to pull my head back onto them with excessive tension in the muscles of the neck?

- Can I feel one side of my body more in contact with the floor than the other side?

- Can I feel tension in either of my legs? Do they want to fall in or out to the sides?

- Can I feel more pressure on the outside or the inside of my feet?

If the answer to any of these questions is 'Yes', the immediate reaction will be to do something to put matters right. The trouble is that anything you do, no matter what, will nearly always increase the muscular tension and make things worse.

According to the Alexander principles, you must try to inhibit any immediate response to your findings and apply conscious thought to help you release tension. In other words you must use your powers of thought alone to let go of any tension that you may feel.

- If your back is arched, then think of the back lengthening and widening. After five minutes or so you may begin to see that your back is becoming flatter as it comes more in contact with the floor.

- If your shoulders are hunched, think of your shoulders going away from your ears. Very soon you will often find that the tension in your shoulder is releasing.

- If your shoulders are curving forward towards each other, think of them going away from each other. This should produce a widening of the upper part of the chest.

- If the books feel hard underneath your head, think of the head going forward and upwards away from your spine. This will ease the muscular tension in the neck so that the chin drops towards the chest.

- If you find that one side of the body is pushing down into the floor, then think of that side of the body releasing away from the floor.

- If either leg wants to fall out, then move the foot of that leg away from the other foot. If either leg wants to fall inwards, then place the foot closer to the other foot. This will ease the tension in the legs. Then think of the knees pointing up to the ceiling.

- If one side of either foot is more in contact with the ground than the other side, then think of the other side having more contact.

Don't expect any instant changes, as releasing muscular tension takes time. Be patient; there will be changes but nature does take time to work.

GETTING UP AGAIN

After about twenty minutes, you should be feeling much more relaxed. Before getting up, pause for a moment or two to work out a less stressful way of rising to your feet. There are many ways of doing this, but one of the best is to roll over onto your stomach and then to go on all fours. Kneel up and then put one foot in front of the other to come back into a standing position.

This may take a little longer than leaping straight up, but it does put less strain on the entire body. This way of rising helps to maintain the length of spine that has been achieved while lying. People with chronic back pain cannot usually get up in any other way.

LENGTHENING THE SPINE

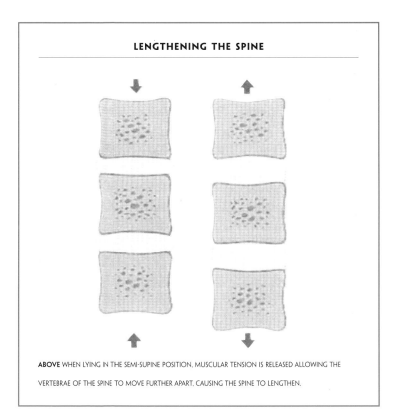

ABOVE WHEN LYING IN THE SEMI-SUPINE POSITION, MUSCULAR TENSION IS RELEASED ALLOWING THE VERTEBRAE OF THE SPINE TO MOVE FURTHER APART, CAUSING THE SPINE TO LENGTHEN.

ANATOMICAL CHANGES AFTER LYING

The spine, or vertebral column, is the main supporting structure of the body. It is made up of a number of bones (vertebrae) that are placed one on top of another. They are separated by sacs of fluid known as the inter-vertebral discs. These discs absorb shock as well as protecting the bones from rubbing against each other during movement. The discs also absorb fluid in order to make the spine longer when movement takes place.

The difference in our height changes between the time we get up in the morning and the time we go to bed at night. We can easily lose an inch or more in height as we go about our normal daily activities. This is entirely due to the loss of fluid from discs that are under stress. This loss is regained while we are asleep at night. It is true, however, that most of this fluid can be regained in only twenty minutes while we are lying down. So if we could lie down for twenty minutes sometime in the afternoon or early evening, then we would lengthen the spine to support us more efficiently for the latter part of the day. We would, therefore, not be so tired at the end of the day and would have more energy to enjoy evening activities. The effect of this is noticeable on people from hotter climates who have siestas; they are able to work into the early hours of the morning without feeling tired.

LEFT THE LENGTH OF THE SPINE IS REDUCED DURING THE COURSE OF A SINGLE DAY. THE SEMI-SUPINE EXERCISE CAN RE-LENGTHEN IT.

THE DECLINE OF STATURE WITH AGE

The loss of fluid from inter-vertebral discs is also connected with a slow loss of height over the years.

Have you ever noticed that your parents or grandparents seem to get shorter, even when you have stopped growing?

A scientist by the name of Junghanns discovered that the size of the inter-vertebral discs does, in fact, get smaller as we get older. This is due to excessive muscular tension building up over the years and pulling the bones of the spine closer together, by as much as two or even three inches.

By lying down for twenty minutes each day you can prevent this from happening. You will not only be easing or preventing serious backache, but you will ensure that the discs in the spine are able to maintain their correct shape for longer. This will help you to move in an easier way, putting less strain on your whole structure.

97

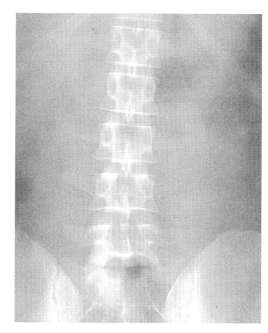

RIGHT THE WAY IN WHICH WE TREAT OUR SPINE DURING OUR LIFETIME, WILL AFFECT HOW IT SERVES US IN OUR LATER YEARS. EXCESSIVE STRAIN AND UNBALANCED MOVEMENT CAN LEAD TO LOSS OF STATURE AND PAIN OR DISCOMFORT.

SQUATTING

Exercise programmes often tend to exercise one set of muscles at the expense of another set. But a simple squat can exercise most of the muscles in the body and yet keep it in perfect balance. It is what children do quite naturally and in many developing countries people carry on doing it into old age. Because of the many hours of sitting that we do, we lose the ability to squat.

If you want to know the correct way to squat, then just watch children of two or three because they are doing it all the time.

When you first start squatting don't overdo it. Start off with small squats, bending your knees and hips just a little. As your legs begin to work so you can go deeper and deeper into the squat. It is easy to overdo it at first so please be gentle with yourself.

As you improve, start to bring the action into your everyday life, such as when bringing the milk out from the fridge or when picking up the post each morning. It may feel most peculiar at first but, after a few weeks, it will feel perfectly normal and your old way will then feel strange.

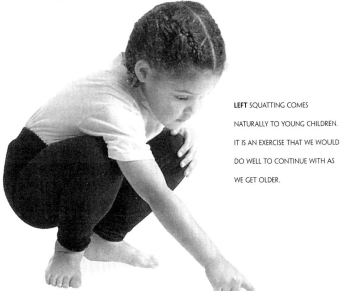

LEFT SQUATTING COMES NATURALLY TO YOUNG CHILDREN. IT IS AN EXERCISE THAT WE WOULD DO WELL TO CONTINUE WITH AS WE GET OLDER.

MIND-WANDERING

Eyes play an important part in the role of body balance and it is important to absorb as much information as possible from what is around you.

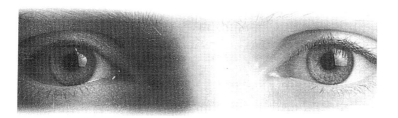

Alexander was convinced that many of our tensions are caused by a lack of interest in the present. He referred to this condition as the 'mind-wandering habit'. Very many people spend much of their lives thinking about what is going to happen or what has happened. This, of course, takes us away from the 'here and now'. Since the eyes are an important for our balance, as well as our sight, then it naturally follows that, if we are thinking about the future or the past while walking or standing, rather than playing attention to whatever we are doing, our whole body balance is going to be affected.

For much of the time we are thinking about something other than what we are doing. Sometimes we will be going upstairs to get something but, by the time we are there, we have forgotten what it was that we went for. Many people often walk past the place they set out for because their minds are thinking about this or that, but not about what they are doing. Have you ever put something of value in a 'safe place', and then forgotten where you put it? The reason why this happens is that you are thinking about other things at the time.

The most common statement that drivers make after an accident is, 'I never even saw him coming.'

This is because, although we go through the movements of looking, we do not actually see what is there.

So this habit of letting our mind wander can be very dangerous as well as time-wasting and inconvenient.

While giving a pupil a lesson, it is possible to feel the muscles tense in order to maintain balance as he or she begins to lose awareness of their surroundings when 'mind-wandering'. Not being in the present will contribute a great deal to the unhappiness caused by the worries and anxieties of modern-day living, because we allow our minds to dwell upon the past, which we cannot change, and the future, which has not yet happened.

IN THE PRESENT

As children we have a natural ability to experience life from moment to moment (the same is true with animals). We are soon, however, encouraged by society to look to the future for our happiness.

Christmas is a good example of this: ten weeks before Christmas arrives, the shops start to fill up with goods that obviously encourage us to dwell on a day that is far ahead in the future.

LEFT YOUNG CHILDREN DO NOT LOOK TO THE FUTURE FOR THEIR HAPPINESS, BUT EXPERIENCE IT IN THE PRESENT.

Many of us look forward to that festive season and yet say after the event,

'I am glad that is over.'

An interesting fact is that more people commit suicide at Christmas than at any other time. In many cases this is due to great disappointment: there is a common thought that if you cannot enjoy yourself at Christmas when can you enjoy yourself?

And what happens on Christmas Day itself? More advertisements on the television, this time about those exotic faraway places, where you can lie in the sun, that will really make you happy!

This is just one example of many that encourage all of us to think about the past or the future – but never to be aware of the present.

It may be said that we have to plan for the future, and I entirely agree, but most of our thoughts can be best described as nonsense. We have not chosen to think these thoughts, our mind has just started to think them without us being aware of what we are thinking.

We start to lose control of our minds in the same way that muscular tension is often out of our control.

The Alexander Technique is a way of directing our conscious minds in order to be more in the present moment. In this way we have the opportunity to be more in tune with nature and to heighten our awareness of the things around us. This will automatically bring more happiness, contentment and peace into our lives.

PREVENTION IS BETTER THAN CURE

Practising the Alexander Technique encourages us to examine every area of our lives to find out what it is that is going wrong. This process takes time. By undoing our mistakes at an early stage, before we begin to experience the symptoms, we can prevent many of our problems.

101

It is, however, easy to become anxious about applying the Technique in our day-to-day lives, even though we may have been shown what to do and even though we know that what we feel may not always be the reality of the situation. This anxiety will only cause tension, which defeats the purpose of the exercise.

If you are patient, however, you will gradually begin to notice changes in the way that you do things. These changes will help the body to perform more efficiently and in a way for which it was designed.

We practise prevention in other areas of our lives; we regularly visit the dentist even when there is no pain; or we have fire and burglar alarms installed. Most of us will have our cars regularly serviced as a precaution against mechanical breakdowns and, in industry, there are many rules and regulations to stop accidents ever taking place. Yet we do not apply the same common-sense principles to our own bodies. A little forethought can often save us much pain or discomfort. So many people could avoid the pain of backache if they took the time to think about the way they used their bodies. If the Alexander Technique was introduced into schools millions of people could be saved the misery of backache.

Lessons

You will save yourself much time and trouble if you have a course of lessons from a qualified teacher. As we have seen, most of us have the problem of faulty perception, and without professional help we can so easily make the problem worse. Not only have teachers had a very extensive training, they are also in a better position to see the cause of your problems.

We, on the other hand, will often try to put things right by expending extra effort, and we will base our efforts on what *feels* right. This is what Alexander experienced and is the very reason why it took him so long to sort out the problem with his voice.

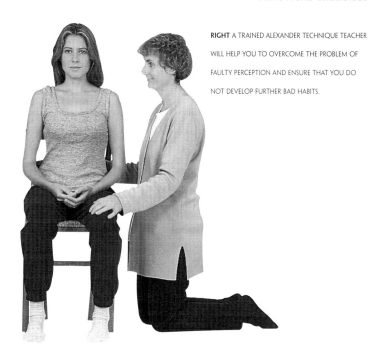

I would like to point out that when your Alexander teacher talks about 'unreliable feelings' he is talking about sensory feelings and not emotions or intuition (a point that has confused many people in the past).

The main trouble with 'doing it yourself' is that many of us do not have a clue where to start. This was the case with me and, even now, I occasionally have one or two lessons to make sure I am not getting into bad habits.

OTHER EXERCISES

There are very few exercise programmes that do not put undue strain on the body; this strain is caused by the same habits of muscular tension and lack of coordination that we use for everything else (perhaps even more so). Even gentle exercises, such as Yoga, can put tremendous stress on the body if they are done without first dealing with the issues of end-gaining and faulty sensory perception. A very famous Yoga teacher from India came to England and, after observing many Yoga classes, asked the instructor why it was that he did not first teach his students to sit, stand and walk with balance and coordination before teaching them the more complicated postures.

Walking, running and swimming are some of the best exercises you can do if you are using yourself in a coordinated manner.

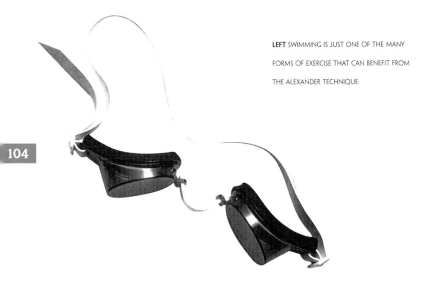

LEFT SWIMMING IS JUST ONE OF THE MANY FORMS OF EXERCISE THAT CAN BENEFIT FROM THE ALEXANDER TECHNIQUE.

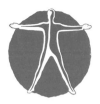

TAKING IT FURTHER

CHAPTER SEVEN

THERE ARE THREE WAYS to learn more about the Alexander Technique:

1. By reading other books.
2. By having Alexander Technique lessons.
3. By attending courses, seminars or workshops.

READING OTHER BOOKS

There are several informative books on the market today, including four by Alexander himself. A list of these books may be found in Further Reading at the end of this chapter.

'Until one is committed there is hesitancy, the chance to draw back, always ineffectiveness, concerning all acts of Initiative and Creation. There is one elementary truth, the ignorance of which kills countless ideas and splendid plans; and the moment one definitely commits oneself, then Providence moves too. All sorts of things occur to help one that would never have occurred. A whole stream of events issues from the decision, raising in one's favour all manner of unforeseen incidents and material assistance that no man could have dreamed would have come his way.'

W.H. MURRAY

ALEXANDER TECHNIQUE LESSONS

Anyone who wants to gain the maximum benefit from Alexander lessons should take a course of individual sessions with a qualified teacher. The number of lessons will vary from pupil to pupil, depending on their initial level of balance and coordination.

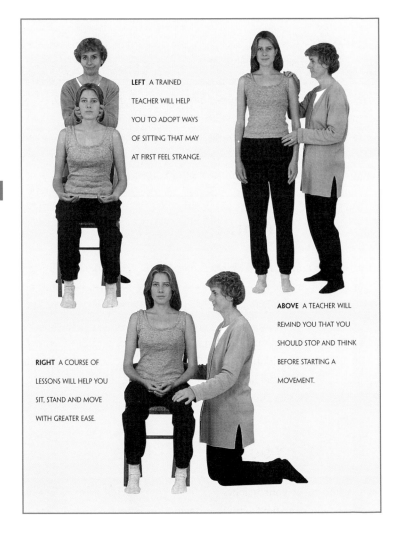

LEFT A TRAINED TEACHER WILL HELP YOU TO ADOPT WAYS OF SITTING THAT MAY AT FIRST FEEL STRANGE.

ABOVE A TEACHER WILL REMIND YOU THAT YOU SHOULD STOP AND THINK BEFORE STARTING A MOVEMENT.

RIGHT A COURSE OF LESSONS WILL HELP YOU SIT, STAND AND MOVE WITH GREATER EASE.

If you already have something wrong with your body you must expect between twenty and thirty lessons.

The length of lessons will vary from teacher to teacher, but the shortest will be half an hour and the longest will be an hour.

COST

The cost of lessons will vary, depending on where you are and how much experience your teacher has had. Lessons will start at around £15.00 and go up to as much as £30.00. If you really cannot afford this payment, then talk it over with your teacher as most will help out if they possibly can.

Lessons may seen very expensive at first, but the combined total is less than what many people spend on a holiday. What you learn in a lesson will stay with you for the rest of you life.

107

FINDING A TEACHER

If you send a stamped addressed envelope to Alexander Technique International or The Society of Teachers of the Alexander Technique, they will send you a list of teachers in your area. You will find a list of societies for various countries at the end of this chapter. All teachers have had similar training, but styles and personalities can differ.

Go by recommendation whenever possible, or have one lesson from three or four teachers. You will find learning easier if you feel happy with your teacher,

YOUR FIRST LESSON

When you meet your teacher for the first time, tell him, or her, as much as you can about why you decided to have lessons. If you are in pain be sure you let the teacher know where it hurts and what position of the body causes the most pain. Also tell him how long ago the problem started. If you have any X-rays of the relevant parts of your body, then bring them along with you. Although the Technique does not deal with specific symptoms, it does help the teacher to know any details that might suggest to them some of your bad habits.

Try to be as relaxed as you can – you have made a positive move to help yourself and now it is important to realize that this process does take time.

WHAT TO WEAR

It is advisable to wear loose, comfortable clothing, although if you have come straight from work this may not be possible and is not essential. You will not be asked to remove any clothing apart from your shoes.

THE FIRST SIX LESSONS

In my experience the first few lessons are sometimes confusing for some people. The teacher will ask you to lie on a table or to sit on a chair while he gently moves your head and limbs. He or she is trying to find areas of tension that may be fixed in your body. When he feels that certain muscles are over-tightened, he will ask you to 'let go' of that tension.

At first you might find it difficult to understand what he is talking about, because most of us are not even aware that these

LEFT LETTING GO OF THE TENSION IN YOUR BODY MAY BE A NEW EXPERIENCE FOR YOU, BUT A TEACHER WILL GUIDE YOU THROUGH.

tensions exist. Lesson by lesson you gradually realize how much tension you have been holding onto. Even then you may find it hard to relax tense muscles as the habits of the muscles may have been with you for a long time.

Little by little you will start to release any unnecessary tension that may have been stored unknowingly for many years.

SUBSEQUENT LESSONS

After you have learnt how to release the tension in muscles that have become shortened, your teacher will take you through some ordinary, everyday activities in order to find out why these particular muscles have become over-tightened.

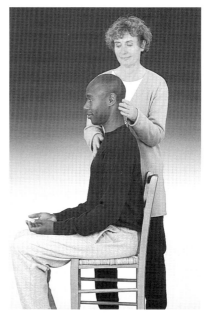

Activities, such as walking, standing, sitting or bending, may have to be learned anew. At first, new ways of performing these actions may feel very strange because we have become so used to moving in our own particular way. If left to ourselves, we would never dream of doing anything that does not 'feel right'.

After a short while the new way of moving begins to feel less strange and sometimes we cannot understand how we could have moved so clumsily for so many years without realizing it.

ABOVE YOUR TEACHER WILL HELP YOU TO RELEARN THOSE EVERYDAY ACTIVITIES THAT, UNTIL NOW, HAVE BEEN CAUSING EXCESSIVE TENSION WITHIN YOUR BODY.

SHORT-TERM EFFECTS
OF AN ALEXANDER LESSON

Even after your very first lesson, you will probably feel much lighter in yourself. Movement can become so much easier and some people describe their experience to be like walking on air or walking on the moon. This is the result of released muscle tension; gravity affects the body in a different way making it much easier to use. At first, this effect may only last for half an hour or so but, as you have more lessons, these feelings of lightness, balance and general ease within your body will last for longer and longer periods. It is then much less effort to carry out many everyday actions.

Immediately after your lessons it is important to take it easy and not rush around as this may undo the teacher's work and the process will take longer to be effective.

It is a good idea not to eat a heavy meal just before having a lesson. It is also best to avoid strenuous exercises if at all possible while undergoing a course of Alexander lessons as this may undo the benefits that the Technique will give you.

PHYSICAL CHANGES

The day after the lesson you may become aware of tensions in some muscles or you may feel an ache where previously you have had no trouble. Do not worry. This is perfectly normal when the body goes through the physical changes that are often brought about by the Alexander Technique. Not everyone experiences them but they are quite common. I remember, after one lesson, feeling as if I had a collar around my neck that prevented me from turning my head (similar to the kind people have to wear after painful neck injuries). I could, of course, turn my head, I was just beginning to realize that I was constantly holding my head with excessive tension.

Because the muscles are being lengthened, you may experience a slight ache in them. This is similar to the growing pains that we have as children and will soon pass.

EMOTIONAL CHANGES

As well as physical changes, you may notice mental or emotional changes. Occasionally, Alexander lessons spark off emotional feelings from childhood: anger, sadness, joy or happiness. Alexander was convinced that every experience we have is transmitted into muscular tension; as you release the tension you may uncover psychological tensions that have been at the bottom of some physical illnesses.

If any changes take place, either physically, mentally or emotionally, be sure to inform your teacher and he or she will be able to help you to understand what is happening.

LONG-TERM EFFECTS OF LESSONS

The long-term effects can be very varied depending on the individual pupil. If you have come with a particular ache or pain, do not expect it to disappear straight away. What is more likely to happen is that the pain will become less intense as the weeks go by until, one day, you wake up and realize that it is not there any more.

In the case of reccurring illnesses, such as migraine or asthma, the attacks often become less frequent as time goes by, and the illness also becomes less severe.

Other physical problems, such as clumsiness or bad posture, can start to improve with time. The effects on the body do take a little while to show themselves and sometimes there will be

RIGHT BAD POSTURE, STANDING WITH THE BODY UNBALANCED AND THE WEIGHT ON ONE LEG, IS THE KIND OF PROBLEM THAT WILL IMPROVE OVER TIME WITH PRACTICE.

periods when you seem to take three steps forward and two backward. Do not worry; many people feel like that.

The main changes will be seen in the long run when you look back, so it is sometimes useful to have photographs taken of yourself just before, and just after, your course of lessons. These will enable you to see the real changes that have taken place.

CHANGING SHAPE

It is often the case that many pupils grow taller or change their shape in some way during lessons, so it is not a good idea to buy shoes or clothes until you are nearing the end of the course of lessons. Many of us hold ourselves in the most distorted positions and when tensions are released the changes can be quite dramatic.

It is common for pupils to grow in height as much as an inch and a half; they appear to lose weight at the same time. This is because most of us have a tendency to 'sink' down into our hips so, by allowing a lengthening of the torso to take place, the pupil can physically become taller and thinner.

BECOMING PEACEFUL

Mental disorders such as anxiety, depression and insomnia can often be helped since freeing our body from all its stresses and strains will naturally affect the mind. Even if you do not have any problems as such, Alexander lessons will probably help you to feel less irritable and not so worried about life in general. I often hear comments such as, 'Since my husband has been involved with the Alexander Technique he is a much nicer man to live with.'

Most people will gain a greater sense of inner peace – something that is very much lacking in this day and age.

Remember, even if you do not have any specific ailments you will still benefit greatly from a course of lessons, perhaps preventing much pain or discomfort later on in life. This is one of the most important insurance policies you could buy.

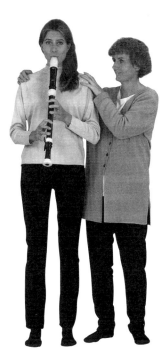

ABOVE A TEACHER WHO SPECIALIZES IN HELPING MUSICIANS MAY BE SUITABLE FOR YOU IF YOU ARE AWARE OF PROBLEMS CAUSED BY PLAYING AN INSTRUMENT.

REGULARITY OF LESSONS

This will be discussed during your first lesson. Very often your teacher may ask you to come twice a week for two or three weeks and then once a week for a further period, which will vary from pupil to pupil. When the Alexander teacher thinks you have grasped the principles of inhibition and direction, he may advise you to come once a fortnight and then once a month.

After the initial course it is advisable to have an occasional lesson every so often as a reminder and a check that you are not falling into any bad habits without realizing it.

113

SPECIAL REQUIREMENTS

If there is a certain activity that you wish to improve, be sure to tell your teacher during your first lesson. Some teachers may specialize in certain sports, while others may have had experience of a particular musical instrument, such as the flute or violin, and therefore may have had similar problems as yourself. Paul Collins, for example, was an Alexander teacher who explored running and himself set ten world records for veterans. He, of course, was an ideal teacher if any sportsmen had running difficulties.

If you cannot find a teacher who is also an expert in your field, do not worry, as any teacher will be able to give you the information that will be required to improve your particular activity.

CHANGE

Alexander once said that people want to change and yet still want to remain the same. By this he meant that many people want to cure a particular problem, or to understand themselves more fully, yet do not want to let go of their habits, especially their mental attitudes to life. Most of what we know has been taught to us as children, and, as children, we have adopted ignorance and prejudices that have become more and more fixed as life goes on.

We have to take lessons with an open mind and a willingness to learn so that we may find out where we are going wrong. If you are able to say, 'I don't know,' then you will be able to learn the Technique so much the quicker. The reason why some people take a long time to learn the Technique is because it is much simpler than they think.

COURSES, SEMINARS OR WORKSHOPS

In my own experience I have found that learning in groups is both economic and a very good way of learning the Technique, especially when you are first starting out. At present I run week-long courses as well as weekend workshops all over Europe. They do not replace individual lessons but in one respect may be even more helpful: seeing another member of the group being shown the basic principles can often make it much clearer to the rest of the group.

To find out about Alexander Technique classes or workshops, ask your local education authority for details, search your local 'what's on' in the newspaper or look at the noticeboard in your library. If you belong to a group of people or a business firm and would like more information on workshops and seminars, both throughout the British Isles and abroad, then please write to me (address in Useful Addresses section). I would be more than happy to receive any invitation to take workshops or to give talks on the subject.

I must stress, however, that if you experience much pain, then individual lessons would be more suitable.

TEACHER QUALIFICATIONS

When you initially approach an Alexander teacher, make sure that he or she has undergone a teachers' training course that is recommended by Alexander Technique International (ATI), or The Society of Alexander Teachers (STAT). A qualified teacher will have undergone a three-year course consisting of fifteen hours a week in college as well as home study. Course work is mainly based around experience but some basic anatomy and physiology is included. All the teachers on the list that ATI and STAT provides are fully qualified.

TRAINING TO BE A TEACHER

When considering whether or not to apply for an Alexander teacher training course you should be aware of the following:

1 Most colleges require a year of continual lessons before applying.

2 There are very few government grants to cover either living expenses or college fees.

3 The fees alone amount to between £10,000 and £15,000 for the three years, payable at the beginning of each year.

4 Courses usually take students in September although some accept students after Christmas and Easter.

5 Many colleges have at least a year's waiting list.

To train as a teacher is physically, mentally and emotionally taxing. You must be sure that it is what you really want to do. Most colleges welcome potential students as observers for a day or two. Addresses of colleges may be found in the Useful Addresses section.

CHAIRS

The wrong sort of chair may be responsible for many of our backaches today. Until quite recently, the Japanese had very few problems with back pain; now it is a problem that is getting rapidly more common. This may well be because our western-type chairs have been introduced into their country.

Recently I wrote a letter to every car manufacturer throughout the world, offering advice on improving car seats. Not one took me up on my offer to know more! Those that did write back stated that they were very happy with their present designs. Unfortunately, this is not the view of many millions of people whose backache is worse after even a short drive.

There are, however, a few chairs on the market that improve posture while sitting. Some of the best are designed and manufactured by John Gorman who has been very interested in the Alexander Technique for many years. He is an engineer who came to study the spine because of his own back pains. His engineering

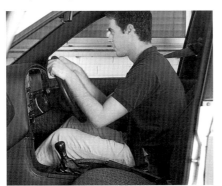

analysis of the problem brought him to many ideas that were very similar to Alexander's in terms of posture and sitting.

LEFT THE DESIGN OF CAR SEATS CAN CAUSE ALL KINDS OF BACK PROBLEMS. LET YOUR TEACHER KNOW IF THIS IS AN AREA WHERE YOU NEED HELP.

One of his first designs was 'the Simple Working Chair', produced in 1984, which has subsequently given comfort to thousands of people. In his two books on the subject he describes the importance of 'good sitting habits' in maintaining a healthy spine and body; his views are similar to those taught by Alexander himself. Mr Gorman has since trained to become a chiropractor.

The basic principle of his chair is that the knees should be below the pelvis, a quite different principle to the design of most chairs. The usual type of chair puts an enormous strain on the spine, back muscles and many of the internal organs. Anyone sitting down for extensive periods (as we all had to do in our school days) would have to tense many of the body's muscles in order to sit up straight. This, in turn, causes the organs, the bones and, ultimately, the entire system to be under stress.

The forward-tilting chair allows the spine and the postural muscles to support and balance the body naturally. You can easily see the effect by placing a telephone book under each of the rear legs of a ordinary kitchen chair. At first, the sensation may seem strange but, after a few minutes, you will appreciate its comfort. The height and angle of the Gorman chairs can be adjusted to suit the individual. Information on these chairs may be obtained from:

John Gorman
Pelvic Posture Ltd
Oaklands
New Mill Lane
Eversley
Hampshire RG27 ORA.

Balance chairs have also attracted a good deal of interest. The forward tilt is admirable but these chairs have a disadvantage: by placing the knees on a pad the feet, with their receptors, are prevented from being placed flat on the floor. Balance chairs are better than conventional chairs but not as beneficial as the Gorman chair.

LAST WORDS

George Orwell once said that, by the time you are forty, you have got the face you deserve. Perhaps the same could be said of our body. If we are using up to five times the energy that we really need to move, then it is hardly surprising that, after a long day, all we can do is 'collapse in a heap'! We have only one body in this life so it is well worth looking after.

As I have already mentioned, the Alexander Technique is not merely a physical technique to improve posture or help eliminate muscle tension that causes pain or discomfort. While it does both of these, it also brings many other benefits. Since the body, mind, emotions and spirit are inseparable, when you release physical tensions throughout your body, your mind and emotions are also affected. As you start to use your body more efficiently, you will in turn have more energy to do the things that you enjoy. Often people who constantly feel tired or drained of energy begin to have more enthusiasm and generally feel more 'alive'. In fact, one of the first things that many people experience after starting Alexander lessons is an improved sleep pattern, and they wake up in the mornings feeling more refreshed. Sleep is the body's natural healing and rejuvenating process, and it is vital for a balanced healthy lifestyle. People's whole attitude to life can change as they begin to look forward to their day rather than wishing their lives away.

It is important to remember that the Technique is not a 'quick fix'. It does take time to learn, and patience and perseverance are the main qualities that you will need during the learning process. Your perseverance will be rewarded, because what you learn during your lessons will be of benefit for the rest of your life.

Through consistent practice of the Alexander Technique you will be able to return to a balanced life where emotions and human values once again have the importance they deserve. This re-balancing will enable you to replace frustration, anxiety and worry with happiness and peace. Concern about the future will gradually be replaced by an enjoyment of each day as it comes, and you will begin to appreciate all the precious gifts that you already possess, rather than hankering for the material goods you have yet to acquire. When you can absorb and enjoy each moment as it comes, then you are truly rich. Your mind can be thinking of experiences of the past or planning the near or distant future, and your emotions can be experiencing the nostalgia of what has gone or longing for what might be, but your body can never leave the here and now. When you focus on it through inhibition and direction you will be able to be truly present, and experience the miracle that each moment brings. Just pause for a moment to consider what is happening in this very instant - your eyes are reading these words, but you are also breathing. The force we call life is causing your lungs to inhale and exhale, giving you life effortlessly. The breath is quietly giving you life, moment by moment, but how often do you really appreciate the miracle of life. With your every breath comes the choice of whether to be unconscious or aware of that miracle. Saint Augustine once said that most people wonder at the heights of mountains, the huge waves in the sea, at the long courses of the rivers or the circular motions of the stars...but they pass by themselves without wondering.

119

As we have seen, The Alexander Technique, is not merely a postural technique to help you to sit, stand and move with poise and grace - it is, in fact, possibly one of the greatest discoveries of the twentieth century, whose great importance is only beginning to emerge. It is a different way of living that allows every one of us to raise our awareness so that we can understand ourselves more fully and be able to claim our supreme inheritance - to be conscious of the limitless potential that resides in each and every one of us and whose power keeps us alive in each and every moment.

I sincerely hope that you have enjoyed this book and found it helpful.

It was written merely as a simple introduction to the Alexander Technique and I hope it has whetted your appetite to find out more. If so, you will find some useful addresses and a further reading list on the next few pages, which will help you to take the next step. So I wish you a happy healthy life and would like to leave you with these thought-provoking words of Henry David Thoreau:

'We must learn to awaken and keep ourselves awake, not by mechanical aids, but by an infinite expectation of the dawn, which does not forsake us in our soundest sleep.

I know of no more encouraging fact than the unquestionable ability of man to elevate his life by a conscious endeavour. It is something to be able to paint a particular picture, or to carve a statue, and so to make a few objects beautiful, but it is far more glorious to carve and paint the very atmosphere and medium through which we look, which morally we can do.

To affect the quality of the day, that is the highest art.'

USEFUL ADDRESSES

Richard Brennan runs a three-year teacher training course in Galway Ireland, as well as shorter weekend and week courses in Ireland, UK, Spain, Greece and the Caribbean. For details of any of these courses send a stamped addressed envelope to:

The Alexander Technique
Training Centre
Richard Brennan
Kirkullen Lodge
Tooreeny
Moycullen, Co Galway
Eire

Alternatively you can visit his website at:
http://homepage.tinet.ie/
~alexander technique

EUROPE
UK
Alexander Technique
International
UK Regional Co-ordinator
66-C Thurlstone Road
London
SE27 0PD

The Society of Teachers of the
Alexander Technique
20 London House
266 Fulham Road
London
SW1O 9EL

DENMARK
The Danish Society of Teachers
of the Alexander Technique
Wergelandsalle 21
DK-2660
Soborg

FRANCE
Alexander Technique
International
French Regional Co-ordinator
10 Rue Froidevaux
Paris
75014

IRELAND

Alexander Technique
International
Irish Regional Co-ordinator
Kirkullen Lodge
Tooreeny
Moycullen, Co Galway
Eire

THE NETHERLANDS

The Netherlands Society of
Teachers of the Alexander
Technique
Max Haverlaarlaan 80
1183 HN Amstelveen

NORWAY

Alexander Technique
International Norwegen
Regional Co-ordinator
Vetrlidsalmenningen 4
5014 Bergen

SWEDEN

Alexander Technique
International
Swedish Regional Co-ordinator
Grundtvigsgatan 9
168 48 Bromma

SWITZERLAND

Alexander Technique
International
Swiss Regional Co-ordinator
Im Theodorshof
Rheinfelden
CH-4310

The Swiss Society of Teachers
of the Alexander Technique
Postfach
CH 8032
Zurich

REST OF THE WORLD
AUSTRALIA

Alexander Technique
International
Australian Regional
Co-ordinator
11/11 Stanley Street
Darlinghurst
NSW 2010

The Australian Society of
Teachers of the Alexander
Technique
PO Box 716
Darlinghurst
NSW 2010

Direction Magazine
(A Journal on the Alexander
Technique with world-wide
subscriptions)
PO Box 276
Bondi
NSW 2026

CANADA
The Canadian Society of
Teachers of the Alexander
Technique
Box 47025
Apt. 12
555 West 12th Avenue
Vancouver
BC V5Z 3XO

SOUTH AFRICA
The South African Society of
Teachers of the Alexander
Technique
35 Thornhill Road
Rondebosch 7700

USA
Alexander Technique
International Inc.(Head Office)
1692 Massachusetts Avenue
3rd Floor
Cambridge
MA 02138

The North American Society of
Teachers of the Alexander
Technique
PO Box 112484
Tacoma
WA 98411-2484

Alexander Technique
Workshops (USA)
PO Box 408
Ojai
California 93024

For all other countries please
contact the country nearest you.

FURTHER READING

Easy-to-follow and informative books on the Alexander Technique:

The Alexander Technique – A Practical Introduction –
Richard Brennan (Element Books 1998)
Mind & Body Stress Relief with the Alexander Technique –
Richard Brennan (Thorsons 1998)
The Alexander Technique Manual – Richard Brennan
(Little Brown 1999)
The Alexander Technique – Chris Stevens (Optima 1987)
Body Learning – Michael Gelb (Aurum Press 1981)
The Principles of The Alexander Technique – Jeremy Chance
(Thorsons 1998)

More in-depth or specialised books on the Alexander Technique:

The Alexander Principle – Wilfred Barlow (Golancz 1973)
The Art of Changing – Glen Park (Ashgrove Press 1989)
Body Awareness in Action – Frank Pierce Jones
(Schocken Books 1976)
F Matthias Alexander – The Man and His Work (Centreline Press 1964)
The Resurrection of the Body – Edward Maisel (Shambala 1969)

Books by Alexander himself, which are sometimes difficult to
follow due to the style of writing:

The Use of the Self – F M Alexander (Gollancz 1985)
Man's Supreme Inheritance – F M Alexander
(Centreline Press 1988)
Conscious Control of the Individual – F M Alexander
(Gollancz 1987)
The Universal Constant in Living – F M Alexander
(Centreline Press 1986)

THE ALEXANDER SELF HELP TAPE

This is the perfect accompaniment to this book and gives clear and concise instructions on:

- How to eliminate unwanted tension.
- How to prevent or relieve back pain.
- How to improve your breathing.
- How to reduce your stress levels.
- How to clear your mind from unwanted thoughts.
- How to practice the two Alexander principles of Inhibition and Direction.
- How to stay in the present moment.

This audio cassette costs £10 (US$20) and is available from:
Richard Brennan, Kirkcullen Lodge, Tooreeny, Moycullen, Co Galway, Eire

INDEX